'This is a book which is long overdue. It is a must-have resource for anyone involved in teaching/facilitating transition to parenting. Written by one of the leading world experts in the field, it serves as both a guide for practice and an academic text with an up-to-date evidence base that addresses a range of different needs in parental terms.'

- Lorna Davies, Ara Institute of Canterbury, Christchurch, New Zealand

T0136327

PARENT EDUCATION FOR THE CRITICAL 1000 DAYS

As research in neuroscience increasingly points to the unparalleled influence of the first 1000 days of life from conception to two years of age in determining the baby's life trajectory, the need for high-quality early parenting education delivered by knowledgeable and dedicated professionals becomes ever more apparent.

This book describes the global aims of early parenting education. It identifies the key areas that research suggests are important: building a relationship with the unborn and newborn baby; preparing for labour and birth; supporting parents' mental health; protecting the couple relationship across the transition to parenthood; and education for special groups such as same-sex couples, women with fear of birth, prisoners, military wives and parents from black and minority ethnic backgrounds.

All practitioners providing early parenting programmes – midwives, health visitors, family link workers, children's centre staff and voluntary sector teachers – will gain new ideas for their practice in this book. Students taking midwifery and early childhood courses will find much to support their studies. Ultimately, the book provides inspiration for all those who are committed to the role of parenting education in reducing social inequalities.

Mary L. Nolan trained as a birth and parenting educator in the UK with the NCT (formerly the National Childbirth Trust). She has taught both parents and educators across the world, and has published extensively in academic, professional and popular journals. Since 2007, she has been Professor of Perinatal Education at the University of Worcester, UK.

PARENT EDUCATION FOR THE CRITICAL 1000 DAYS

Mary L. Nolan

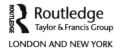
Routledge
Taylor & Francis Group

LONDON AND NEW YORK

First published 2020
by Routledge
2 Park Square, Milton Park, Abingdon, Oxon OX14 4RN

and by Routledge
52 Vanderbilt Avenue, New York, NY 10017

Routledge is an imprint of the Taylor & Francis Group, an informa business

British Library Cataloguing-in-Publication Data
A catalogue record for this book is available from the British Library

Library of Congress Cataloging-in-Publication Data
A catalog record has been requested for this book

ISBN: 978-0-367-42036-9 (hbk)
ISBN: 978-0-367-44540-9 (pbk)
ISBN: 978-0-367-81749-7 (ebk)

Typeset in Interstate
by Newgen Publishing UK

This book is dedicated, with immense gratitude, to my husband, whose unfailing interest and support underpin it.

CONTENTS

1 Introduction 1

2 Aims of early parenting education 6

3 Effective parent educators: skills and relationships 21

4 Supporting parents' prenatal relationship with their baby 34

5 Stress and relaxation: education for a calm pregnancy 42

6 Education and support for normal birth 55

7 Education and support for home birth 72

8 Education and support for women with fear of childbirth 84

9 Debriefing women following childbirth: birth story workshops 97

10 Education and support for fathers 104

11 Education and support for the couple relationship across the transition to parenthood 119

12 Education and support for same-sex couples 129

13 Education and support for interacting with the baby: emotional regulation and relationship learning 135

14 Education and support for breastfeeding 147

15 Education and support for young mothers 160

16 Education and support for mothers and fathers in prison   174

17 Education and support for at-home parents in military families   184

18 A note on education and support for parents of twins   192

19 A note on early parenting education for mothers and fathers
    from minority communities   197

20 The way forward: preconception education and support   203

    Appendix: Teaching and learning activities   207

    Index   234

1   Introduction

When I started work as a childbirth educator in the 1980s, I ran *classes*. This was long before Cliff and Deery's article, 'Too much like school: Social class, age, marital status and attendance/non-attendance at antenatal classes', helped us understand that the word 'classes' is negatively loaded for many parents. My classes focused on the discomforts of late pregnancy and how to manage them, preparation for labour and birth and a little on breastfeeding. I ran eight-week courses which were well attended and there was plenty of time to share knowledge, ideas and feelings and to support parents to make informed choices about their care. There was also a strong focus on practising skills for coping with the intensity of contractions in labour. Every class would include the opportunity to try out different positions, practise calm breathing and experience massage. Even in the 1980s, the alienation of women from their bodies owing to several decades of increasingly rigid medical control of birth was a challenge for educators seeking to build parents' self-efficacy for labour and birth.

I enjoyed leading the classes very much and I think the people who came enjoyed them too (by and large!). The 1990s, however, changed the antenatal curriculum for ever. This was the decade of the brain and our understanding of how the baby's brain (not just her body) develops in the womb, and the factors that impact development, grew massively. We learnt that stress experienced by the mother is felt by her baby as well, and if she is living with unrelenting, severe stress, it is likely that her baby will be born prematurely, and with his stress thermometer set much too high – perhaps for the rest of his life.

What we didn't know, and still don't, is how much maternal stress is 'too much' for the baby. However, it certainly makes sense that maternal stress hormones will pass to the baby and that nature might make a judgement, based on the level of those hormones, about the kind of environment the baby will have to survive in after birth. If the extra-uterine environment is 'read' by the baby in utero as dangerous, nature might sensibly provide the new baby and growing child with a hair-trigger response to every perceived threat; if the extra-uterine environment is read as benign, nature might prepare the baby to be less anxious and more relaxed about the world.

During the 1990s and noughties, knowledge of what was happening in the womb grew exponentially and, very soon, it was being posited that babies' entire futures, from birth to old age, were shaped by their 'experiences' inside the mother. Successful (or unsuccessful) functioning as an adult was being traced back, at least in part, to the nine months spent in the womb.

Families were changing, too. The traditional nuclear family, comprising married parents and the children of that marriage, was now a minority situation; new family structures – more complex than previously – were being created, offering babies and small children different 'environments of relationships' in which to grow up. The baby might be born into a blended family where one or both parents had children from previous relationships; or into a family where his principal carers were two women or two men; or into a single-parent family, whether a mother or a father.

The relationship between the baby's parents was, at the start of the 21st century, increasingly recognised as playing a significant part in the way in which the child developed emotionally and socially. Stress between parents was identified as affecting children; some children would cope well with their parents' unhappiness, but others, perhaps the majority, would find such stress frightening and respond either by withdrawing into themselves, or by manifesting aggressive, non-compliant behaviours. The mental health of the mother was also very much to the fore. Research had demonstrated that the babies of depressed mothers who were unable to communicate with them in a normal, healthy way – by making eye contact and responding to their cues – were likely to have poor mental health themselves, with boys often more seriously impacted than girls. In recent years, paternal mental health has at long last been recognised as also profoundly influential in the life of the baby and young child. A father who is depressed because his partner is depressed, or because of the upheaval in every aspect of his life occasioned by the arrival of the baby, or who is suffering from posttraumatic stress disorder after being present at a difficult birth will be unable to make a positive contribution to the environment in which his child is growing up.

Most families, given enough support and sufficient income, cope with the changes that a new baby brings, even though there is probably no family which doesn't experience challenges along the way, and periods of disorientation and distress. However, as the present century has advanced, the need to give extra education and support to families struggling with poverty and other stressors has been increasingly recognised. Research has revealed the way in which such families negatively impact children's life chances – in school, in employment and in relationships. The new science of epigenetics, although in its infancy, is strongly suggesting the possibility of *inter-generational* transmission of disadvantage, and the drive for 'early intervention' to break into the cycle of disadvantage at the very start of a baby's life has gained momentum.

Such research has been a powerful motivator for many countries to put what is now called 'the critical 1000 days' on to the political agenda. At EU level, it has been accepted that parenting support should be mainstreamed in political consciousness. This means paying attention not only to education for parenthood, but also to ensuring that social security arrangements, healthcare, housing and the media are all supportive of young families. COFACE Families Europe, a pluralistic network of civil society associations representing the interests of all families, describes the need for:

> policies and legislation that impact the lives of children and families, in particular in the fields of social protection and inclusion ... prevention of and fighting child poverty, reconciling family and work life, migration, inclusive education and early childhood education and care, and parenting support services to families.

(www.coface-eu.org/)

Given the implicit 'call to arms' from the research community, new social structures and a new political commitment to early family life, the way in which women and men were prepared for the arrival of a new baby in the 21st century had to be updated, made more relevant and better able to help them anticipate and meet the challenges of the *transition to parenthood*, rather than focusing solely on labour, as had been the essence of antenatal education in the 1970s, '80s and '90s. Preparation for labour and birth remained, of course, important. In a world where the media portrayed (and continues to portray) birth as dramatic and dangerous, often requiring heroic medical intervention to save the life of mother and baby, women were, at the start of the 21st century, approaching labour with at least as much trepidation as their 19th-century sisters who feared, with justification, that they might die in childbirth. Keeping birth – *normal vaginal birth* – on the antenatal education agenda was vital because research was starting to demonstrate that babies benefitted, in ways not previously understood, from being born vaginally. The baby's microbiome (which shapes his lifetime health) was, it was discovered, most effectively seeded by the baby having contact with the mother's vaginal flora during the act of birth. Therefore, as the caesarean section rate soared, the need to support women and their partners to believe in their ability to have a straightforward vaginal birth, and to educate them in how to work with the woman's body during labour, was as great as it had ever been.

But antenatal education had to be much broader than it had been in the 1980s. The 'teachable moment' of pregnancy when human beings are specially motivated to reflect on their lives, on who they are and what they aspire to be, on what they want for their babies and how they might achieve success and happiness for them, demanded a richer educational agenda than educators had provided previously. Now, we wanted to offer parents the precious opportunity, within a safe group of peers, to look at their mental health, their relationships and how to make decisions about parenting in the very complex world their babies were being born into. Educators like myself also wanted to move well away from a deficit model of parenting that focused on what parents *shouldn't* do, to a model of loving, respectful relationships between parents and their baby. We wanted to be realistic about the challenges of caring for a baby while celebrating the joys of early parenting. While the research was pointing to the benefits for *society* of ensuring that children have a great start in life, educators wanted to support positive parenting because children *deserve* to have cuddles, hugs, conversations, nutritious food and exercise.

The ongoing challenge for early parent educators of synthesising research and new social frameworks into a dynamic, relevant parent education agenda is incredibly exciting. What do parents-to-be want to know about? When do they need to know it? What skills would they like to acquire? When? How do they want to learn? What kinds of transition to parenthood groups provide the best education and support?

There is a cacophony of voices in the parent education arena. Where antenatal classes focusing on labour and birth were traditionally led by midwives, health visitors and lay teachers trained by the National Childbirth Trust, the new broader agenda for early parenting education has brought new educators to the fore who feel they can offer insights and expertise valuable to parents. Staff in children's centres, parent link workers, nursery nurses and private individuals now provide antenatal and postnatal education and support. No single professional group and no single service can any longer claim a monopoly of wisdom that enables them to provide front-line education for families across the transition to parenthood. Territorialism in parent education is no longer appropriate; ensuring a high standard is. This book hopes to make a contribution towards ensuring the quality of early parenting education.

With so many educators in the field, it is all the more important that educators are clear about their aims, what it is we hope to achieve and how we intend to achieve it. We need to understand the topics that parents say are most helpful to them and how they want to learn, what individuals in different circumstances need in preparation for parenting, and how those needs can be met sensitively without prejudice, intended or otherwise, on the part of the educator.

This book aims to strengthen the confidence, knowledge and skills of those committed people who are working in the very early years with mothers, fathers and families as they make the transition to parenthood. It aspires to help educators understand what they can do to ensure that all babies have the best possible start in life, and spend their first years in an environment that nurtures them and optimises their potential. It aims to do what it can to level the playing field for children at the start of life by supporting educators to assist *all* parents to provide an optimal home learning and home nurturing environment. It sees parent education in pregnancy and the early postnatal period as an essential component of the 'action' that Michael Marmot spoke about in his seminal report (2010:20) on health inequalities in the UK: 'Action to reduce health inequalities must start before birth and be followed through the life of the child. Only then can the close links between early disadvantage and poor outcomes throughout life be broken.' This book is about reducing health inequalities through early parenting education that builds the confidence of parents-to-be and new parents, and their knowledge and skills to be the excellent parents that they so eagerly desire to be. It firmly believes that investing early is investing wisely.

References

Cliff, D., Deery, R. (1997) Too much like school: Social class, age, marital status and attendance/non-attendance at antenatal classes. *Midwifery*, 13(3):139–145.

COFACE Families Europe (2016) Available at: www.coface-eu.org/about-2/what-is-coface-families-europe/ (accessed 12 November 2019).

Marmot, M., Goldblatt, P., Allen, J., Boyce, T., McNeish, D. et al. (2010) *Fair Society, Healthy Lives*. London: The Marmot Review.

2 Aims of early parenting education

Parenting interventions may reduce health inequalities across the social gradient if they result in:

- *More parents with good mental health, including in pregnancy*
- *More children with secure attachment – more parents engaging positively with, and actively listening to, their children*
- *An increase in the number and frequency of parents regularly talking to their children...and reading to their children every day*
- *Improved cognitive, social and emotional, language and physical health outcomes for children.*

(Public Health England 2014:4)

For at least two centuries, 'experts' (e.g. L. Emmett Holt, G. Stanley Hall, John Watson, Dr Spock, Anna Freud, T. Berry Brazelton, Maggie Myles), doctors, nurses, midwives, women's rights activists and lay teachers have supported the provision of early parenting education in the belief that it is valuable in helping women and men achieve greater enjoyment of parenting, and better outcomes in all aspects of life for their children. This persistent belief in the value of parenting education for the 'critical 1000 days' from pregnancy to two years of age should induce both a sense of humility in contemporary educators (we are certainly not the first to have walked this path) and confidence that, for many years, passionate campaigners, researchers and practitioners have seen the potential of early parenting education to make a difference to children's lives.

Delivering any kind of education, to any group of people, demands that the educators should be clear about what it is that they are trying to achieve. Without having established the direction of travel to their own satisfaction, the sessions they lead will be rudderless, and while they might be entertaining, and even informative, they are unlikely to contribute to any coherent strategy for improving the cognitive, social and emotional wellbeing of the individuals who participate.

Institutions that provide early parenting education, whether they be health or social welfare organisations, businesses or charities, must know what their aims are for the educational interventions to which they commit staff, time and resources. They may need to rely on programmes that do not have a strong evidence base, whether because no research is available, or because studies that have been carried out are of poor quality, or because they have chosen to devise their own programmes for their particular clientele, rather than use existing ones. This is all the more reason for institutions and individuals to be clear about their aims and the theoretical mechanisms by which they think the programme will be effective.

The transition to parenthood has been described as 'a teachable moment'. Expectant and new parents are especially open to reflecting on their lifestyles and making healthy changes, and to learning new information and practising skills to help them care for their baby (Feinberg & Kan, 2008; Sher, 2016). Therefore, practitioners providing education at this critical period have both an exceptional opportunity and an exceptional responsibility.

Over forty years ago...

In 1976, Steven Schlossman noted that:

> *Parent education to upgrade child-care practices in the home shows signs of becoming the pet educational reform of the 1970s.*
>
> (Schlossman 1976:436)

While Schlossman goes on to demonstrate that early parenting education in the USA had, in fact, a long history prior to the 1970s, he himself was highly sceptical that it could achieve the aims that policy makers and practitioners aspired to. Nevertheless, his observation that it would become a key player in interventions to support family life has been borne out over the last four decades.

Two years later, in a paper entitled 'Towards improvements in parenting', Smith and Smith (1978) noted that many parents felt unprepared for the realities of looking after a baby and the responsibilities of new parenthood, and that there was a dearth of parent education programmes to which they could turn for information and support. The particular prenatal/postnatal programme on which they reported had, as its aims:

- To prepare parents to meet new challenges
- To promote healthy parent–child relationships
- To promote independence and confidence in problem solving by parents
- To establish and strengthen parents' systems of support (p22)

The authors also expressed their vision that early parenting education should be 'a first step towards a preventative approach to health' (p27), an aspiration that was to move centre-stage as understanding of the inter-generational transmission of disadvantage and poor parenting started to be elucidated by neuroscience and developmental psychology in the 1990s.

In the late 1970s, Burton-White's influential book, entitled, *The First Three Years of Life* (1978), regretted the limited availability of preparation and support for parenthood and agreed with Smith and Smith that early parenting education was an important preventative measure. Waiting to intervene until the child was two years old was 'already much too late' (p5), as:

> *In their simple everyday activities, infants and toddlers form the foundations of all later development.*

(pix)

These late-20th-century advocates for early parenting education saw it as a primary prevention strategy and as an important early intervention for improving outcomes for children. In 1974, Bronfenbrenner (1974:1) noted that early intervention was 'a strategy for counteracting the destructive effects of poverty on human development'. He argued that 'early' must mean in the first year of life because the sooner the mother and baby entered into reciprocal communication, the better the outcomes for the child.

The 'decade of the brain' in the 1990s threw new light on brain development in unborn and newborn babies, and further stimulated interest in the potential of transition to parenthood education. At the beginning of the 21st century, the 'critical 1000 days' became (and remains) a global catch phrase, enshrining a new understanding that, while genetics may determine a child's characteristics and potential, it is the environment that determines the extent to which these are expressed and realised. For unborn babies and very young children, the 'environment' is primarily shaped by their relationship with their key carers and the relationship between the carers themselves. Therefore, the overarching aim of transition to parenthood education is to intervene early to support parents to provide as sensitive an environment of relationships as possible in order to influence the present and future mental health and wellbeing of their children. As the first years of parenting often determine later parenting (Gutman et al., 2009), early intervention would logically provide better and longer-lasting outcomes for children (Molinuevo, 2013). Positive collateral from improving early childhood includes fewer demands when children are older on a variety of services such as education, social security, healthcare and the judiciary (WAVE Trust, 2013:6). *Social Justice Begins with Babies* (Scottish Coalition, 2014) succinctly summarises the significance of early intervention:

> *Although later interventions can be very helpful, there is no second chance to make a good first impression on the brains, bodies and behaviours of babies and toddlers.*

(p2)

Effectiveness of early parenting education

While research into the impact of early parenting education remains inconclusive, the 2007 Cochrane review, 'Individual or group antenatal education for child-birth or parenthood, or both', also acknowledges that the quality of studies is generally poor.

> *There are many varied ways of providing ... antenatal education and some may be more effective than others. The review found 9 trials involving 2284 women. Interventions varied greatly and no consistent outcomes were measured. The review of trials found a lack of high quality evidence from trials and so the effects of antenatal education remain largely unknown.*
>
> (Gagnon & Sandall 2007:Abstract)

In considering the impact of education on parenting skills, the review looked solely at education provided in pregnancy; its remit was not to look at education provided both prenatally and postnatally, or just postnatally. Additionally, it looked only at outcomes of antenatal education for women, rather than for fathers, partners and families. It concluded by calling for further research.

Gilmer et al. (2016:118) also found, in their examination of parent education interventions designed to support the transition to parenthood, that there is 'no compelling evidence to suggest that a single educational programme or delivery format [is] effective at a universal level'. However, they also highlighted serious deficiencies in the research and concluded that:

> *The importance of the transition to parenthood and its impact on parent and child wellbeing warrant careful consideration of current programming and careful evaluation of future initiatives.*
>
> (Gilmer et al. 2016:119)

Neither of these reviews, therefore, should dent the persistent belief in the value of parent education which is shared by parents themselves along with parent-focused charities, health and social care professionals and government and its agencies. Human beings are pre-eminently learning animals, programmed to seek information, to acquire skills and to devise strategies for coping with new experiences based on learning acquired from previous experiences. To seek parenting education responds to the evolutionary drive to protect the next generation as best we can.

This book acknowledges wholeheartedly that early parenting education may be a *necessary* condition of positive parenting while not being a *sufficient* one. To argue that it is *necessary* may seem surprising – but it should be borne in mind that there has always been parent education. Historically, this has been in the form of an 'apprenticeship' system. Down the centuries, pre-adolescent and adolescent girls learned about giving birth and caring for babies from their own mothers, and boys learned about fathering from their fathers. In the 21st century in post-industrial countries, early parenting education may be considered *necessary* because involvement in the care and nurture of very young children is an experience that fewer and fewer women and men have had by the time they come to adulthood. This should encourage educators in their work while stimulating governments at regional, national and international levels, to enhance its impact through measures that meet the *sufficiency* requirement. Parent education programmes must be part of a broader sweep of measures (affordable housing, adequately paid employment, access to safe environments and leisure opportunities) that ensure parents have the financial and emotional resources to give their children the warm, positive parenting that is their right.

Universal early parenting education

The most rigorous studies of parent education have been directed at programmes designed for especially vulnerable families. Many programmes targeted at families in the greatest need, such as Family Foundations created by Mark Feinberg in the USA and the Family Nurse Partnership created by David Olds, also in the USA, are manualised and therefore lend themselves to being evaluated using robust measures such as randomised controlled trials. It is far harder to assess the impact of early parenting education programmes that are offered on a universal basis to participants from immensely varied backgrounds. The number of confounding factors in assessing the impact of such programmes is infinite. Yet there are excellent arguments for universal early parenting education programmes:

> First, they can improve mental well-being at population level. Second, they are less stigmatising. Third, universal practices can address problems before they reach clinical levels.

> (Molinuevo 2013:44)

Universal-level programmes may be able to identify and help parents find solutions to problems before families require more intensive support at far greater cost to the national purse. They have the potential to improve parents' mental health, and therefore, their children's, at population level and can disseminate understanding of positive parenting as widely as possible so that it becomes part of the received culture of parenting. Targeted programmes aim to support families where there is perceived to be a risk of child neglect or abuse, but most abuse is, in fact, unpredictable and, like domestic violence, is more frequent, if not more prevalent, in the larger part of the population which is not apparently at risk. Therefore, commitment to a universal service of preparation for parenting can be an important component of child protection.

This book is about the aims, content and process of *universal* early parenting education. It believes that a universal offer normalises parent education so that women and men see it as an everyday part of preparation for having a baby and making a successful transition to new parenthood.

Aims of early parenting education

To increase self-efficacy for labour and birth

Women's and men's first engagement with family services is often at the time of a first pregnancy when they come into contact with the maternity service. The nature of that contact – whether respectful and compassionate or dismissive and uncaring – may determine whether they engage with other family-orientated services in the future. Giving birth is a life-transforming event with immense implications for women's physical and psychological wellbeing, and for their partners' mental health also. The way in which parents are affected – for better or for worse – by their experience of labour is critical in influencing how their baby will experience the first weeks of life. Therefore, early parenting education must include preparation for labour and birth as this is the pivotal event in the formation of a new or extended family.

It is a subject for debate amongst childbirth educators as to whether education in the antenatal period should focus exclusively on straightforward vaginal birth with no information being provided about pharmacological forms of pain relief, assisted birth or caesarean section, or whether time should be devoted to all of these interventions, given the frequency with which women experience them. The concern is that, by including information about and discussion of interventions, the impression may be conveyed that these are a 'normal' part of having a baby in affluent 21st-century countries. However, if antenatal sessions cover only the events of a straightforward vaginal birth, might this risk leaving women and their birth companions unprepared for eventualities that are common in maternity units, and potentially traumatised as a result?

The caesarean section rate in the UK has been climbing over the last 30 years, from 12% in 1990 (Parliamentary Office of Science and Technology, 2002) to 28% in May 2017 (NHS Digital, 2017). Yet birth without interventions has many benefits for women's physical and mental health, and for maternity services in terms of reduced expenditure (O'Mahoney et al., 2010; Kassebaum et al., 2014; Smith et al., 2016). There is also evidence that women themselves would like to labour without drugs or medical interventions (Care Quality Commission, 2015; Wharton et al., 2017).

Anecdotal evidence would suggest that women and their partners are keen to receive information about pharmacological pain relief and the interventions available in hospital during labour. However, if self-efficacy for normal birth is to be strengthened, antenatal education needs to increase understanding of the *normal* progress of labour, of how the woman's body works to birth her baby and of the cognitive and physical strategies that women and their partners can employ to cooperate with the natural birthing process. Building self-efficacy for normal labour and birth is a central aim of early parenting education and contributes to an ecology of normal birth that protects human wellbeing and reduces dependence on expensive and finite healthcare resources.

To improve sensitivity to infants

Early parenting education aims to help mothers and fathers establish an enduring emotional relationship with their child, based on frequent, reciprocal, sensitive and enjoyable interactions. Many children do not have a secure attachment to one or more significant adults in their lives. Around one in four children avoid their parents when distressed because they have learned that their parents ignore their needs, and a further 15% actively resist their parents because they are the cause of their distress, rather than the means by which it is resolved (Moeller et al., 2013). Sadly, the legacy of poor early attachment is felt down the generations as insecure attachment affects the kind of relationships children form when adults, and the way in which they themselves parent (Sher, 2016). Parenting education programmes may contribute to secure attachment by building the relationship between the mother and father/partner with their unborn and newborn baby, and supporting parents to be mind-minded, that is to see their young child as a unique individual with her own mind, rather than as a (mere) entity with (primarily) physical needs. By increasing parents' understanding of their young children, and their ability to interact positively with them, early parenting education promotes an 'overall enjoyment of parenting roles' (Moeller et al., 2013:430), and more confident and responsive parenting.

To enhance practical parenting skills

In an era when many parents in wealthy, post-industrial, 'minority' countries know little or nothing about how to care for a baby, parents are increasingly anxious about everyday babycare (The Scottish Government, 2012a). Education provided across the transition to parenthood therefore aims to enhance competence in the essential parenting skills of feeding, soothing, dressing and bathing babies, by sharing information and developing skills to enable parents to meet their baby's basic physical needs. Education also brings parents' attention to the opportunities provided by essential babycare tasks to communicate with the baby through stroking, mutual gaze, talking and singing. Fathers in particular want and benefit from learning how to look after their baby as having these skills enables them to find 'a way in' to a relationship with their baby during the first weeks of life, especially if the mother is breastfeeding.

To reduce parental stress and support mental health

Uncontrolled parental stress affects every aspect of family life – parents' relationship with their baby, with each other and with wider family and friendship networks – as well as their ability to cope with everyday parenting challenges. Relentless stress may compromise the baby's physical safety as well as his or her emotional wellbeing if stress manifests as aggression (Lieberman & Van Horn, 2013). A primary cause of stress is poverty and the quality of parenting of mothers on low incomes has been shown to be more threatened than that of mothers buffered by an adequate secure income (Gutman et al., 2009).

It was reported in 2014 by the London School of Economics and Centre for Mental Health that the total economic and social long-term cost of perinatal mental health problems is around £8.1 billion for each one-year cohort of births in the UK (Maternal Mental Health Alliance, 2014). In the short term, mental ill health impacts the quality of life of the mother, and therefore of her baby and other family members, and in the long term it increases the likelihood of problems developing in her child that persist into adulthood. Early parenting education can aim to reduce this immediate and longer-term suffering in two ways. Some mothers who are anxious or depressed antenatally will be helped by support mediated by friendships made at parent education sessions. Early parenting education can help parents to identify the signs of mental illness and encourage them to seek help as soon as possible. Even if this impacts the mental wellbeing of only a small number of mothers, the concomitant reduction in demand on health and social care services will mean a considerable reduction in expenditure. *Fathers'* poor mental health also adversely impacts young children, including the development of emotional and behavioural problems, and unsatisfactory peer relationships. Domoney et al. (2013) argue that providing information about the possible difficulties of becoming a father can help to normalise men's experiences and encourage disclosure of problems early on.

To strengthen the couple relationship across the transition to parenthood

The transition to first-time parenthood is difficult for many couples (Doss et al., 2009). They may struggle with exhaustion, role overload and reduced time for intimacy and to participate in previously enjoyed leisure activities. Tiredness exacerbated by feeling overwhelmed with responsibility may lead to failures of communication (Howard & Brooks-Gunn, 2009) and decreasing support for each other.

Conflict between parents impacts children's health and wellbeing (Glade et al., 2005):

> *The quality of the interparental relationship, specifically how parents communicate and relate to each other, is increasingly recognised as a <u>primary</u> influence on effective parenting practices and children's long-term mental health and future life chances.*
>
> (Early Intervention Foundation 2019)

Children base their own relationships on a template that is laid down during infancy as a result of observing and being affected by the relationship between their key carers, generally their mother and father:

> *The more respectful and communicative the relationships [children] experience early in life, the more positive their own relationships are likely to be in later life and possible future parenthood.*
>
> (The Scottish Government 2012b:33)

It is therefore an aim of early parenting education to strengthen the couple relationship in the antenatal period and enable partners to anticipate catalysts for dissatisfaction following the birth, such as differences of opinion about how to care for the baby, and who should be responsible for which babycare and household tasks (Waliski et al., 2012).

To build social support

Social support has been defined as the interpersonal resources that individuals can access when they are faced with the inevitable stresses and strains of everyday life (McVeigh, 2000:26). The importance of social support in protecting individuals' wellbeing has long been recognised:

> *Increasing the supportiveness of individuals' social environments is becoming a central focus in the prevention of pathology and the promotion of personal well-being.*
>
> (Mitchell et al. 1982:77)

However, the decline of family and community networks in minority countries means that new parents may find themselves experiencing a reduction in the number and quality of social interactions that they can enjoy following the birth of a child, and especially a first child (Vimpani, 2001). This shrinking of the social network occurs at exactly the time when it is most needed (Scott et al., 2001). As long ago as 1974, Bronfenbrenner suggested that enabling mothers to meet in a group could provide mutual reinforcement and a source of security. Parent-to-parent support appears to play a key role in promoting social and emotional wellbeing for families (Moeller et al., 2013:435) and belonging to peer support groups is rated highly by most parents (The Scottish Government, 2012:28).

Lack of social support has been found to correlate with poor parenting quality, child physical and emotional abuse and maternal depression (Scott et al., 2001). Gutman et al. (2009) note that mothers who have better social networks have more positive interactions with their babies and suggest that this may be due to improved maternal mental health as a result of the support they are able to access. McVeigh (2000) notes a connection between mothers participating in community activities outside the home and engaging in self-care activities.

Hanna et al. (2002) argue that building or enhancing mothers' and fathers' social support network following the birth of a baby should be seen as a primary prevention strategy in mediating the impact of stress on health and parenting practices. Such networks enable parents to share responses to common childcare problems, and to develop a sense of agency that they can achieve their goals for their baby and family.

To build strong, healthy communities

Supporting and educating parents of young children is a primary means of building a culture of health and creating stability in communities as these are dependent in large part on the wellbeing of families (Verbiest et al., 2016:4). Stable families contribute to stable communities which can provide security and opportunities for all their members, and enable parents to feel optimistic about their children's future (Moeller et al., 2013:430). The Scottish *National Parenting Strategy* (The Scottish Government, 2012b) notes the link between deprivation and poor literacy, and the link between poor literacy and community decline, and aims to enrich community life through parent education which includes a focus on encouraging and supporting parents to read to their babies and toddlers.

To ameliorate social inequalities

It has long been the aspiration of parent education to 'level the playing field' by helping children born into under-privileged families to enjoy the same degree of physical, emotional and cognitive wellbeing as children born into easier circumstances, and therefore to have as good a chance of leading a healthy and rewarding life, and enjoying financial security. Early childhood is critical for health equity (Braveman et al., 2018). Verbiest et al. (2016) note that the baby's life trajectory may be determined by the health and socio-economic circumstances of his or her parents, while Scotland's *National Parenting Strategy* (The Scottish Government, 2012b) claims that the most significant influence on a child's educational attainment and employment opportunities is the way in which she or he was parented. Donkin et al. (2014:89) describe the aim of early parenting education as 'to flatten the social gradient'. In their opinion, one of the means through which this can be achieved is by:

> *Improving parenting skills ... by communicating 'what works' to all parents, with interventions available to those who might be at most risk.*

Gutman and Feinstein (2010:555) argue that disadvantaged children are more likely to do well if they receive 'involved, engaged parenting' and therefore, that parent education programmes which help parents to interact sensitively with their babies and toddlers, and to provide a rich home learning environment, will foster the positive development of less privileged children, so reducing inequalities dependent on social circumstances. Kiernan and Mensah (2011) agree, stating that positive parenting contributes to school achievement and is a mediator in reducing the effects of poverty and disadvantage. Early parenting education and support should therefore be seen as a social investment (Molinuevo, 2013) and as a means of achieving social justice (Sher, 2016).

Conclusion: early parenting education – necessary but not sufficient

The potential of early parenting education has been conceptualised for at least the last 40 years at all levels of Bronfenbrenner's ecological model (Figure 2.1). It has been seen as having the capacity to influence the microsystem, namely the healthy development of the child; the mesosystem – the relationship between the people responsible for the baby's care; the exosystem – the way in which early parenting is affected by social networks; the macrosystem – the biological embedding of social adversity or privilege through the home learning environment; and the chronosystem – the way in which disadvantage is transmitted across generations.

The provision of early parenting education to all parents is one means of ensuring that every child has the best possible start in life. However, parenting programmes are *not* a magic bullet (Public Health England, 2014:28). They cannot be expected to remedy all social ills. They are one strategy for improving outcomes for children across the life trajectory, but they cannot achieve this without a raft of other strategies to support new families.

The single most important, broad risk factor that predicts later maladjustment is poverty since this amplifies and concentrates all the other risks (Brooks-Gunn et al., 2000). Parents living in poverty and engaging in the unhealthy behaviours that sometimes accompany it, such as drug and alcohol abuse, may demonstrate poor parenting in many different domains. They may be unable to provide responsive, warm relationships, a stimulating learning and play environment, a nourishing diet and security in the form of routines around sleeping, eating and going out:

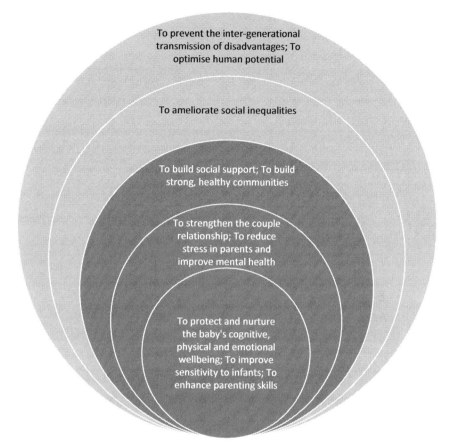

Figure 2.1 Aims of early parenting education and support, reflecting Bronfenbrenner's ecological system – microsystem, mesosystem, endosystem, exosystem, chronosystem.

The dark grey segments capture the aims of high-quality universal parent education at the level of the family and community; the light grey segments are the broader social aims.

> *When families are disadvantaged, disruption to parenting is not specific to any particular parenting behaviour, but may impact negatively across many aspects of parenting.*
>
> (Kiernan & Mensah 2011:328)

Nobody is likely to argue that bringing up children with limited resources makes parenting easier. It has been noted that the drudgery of poverty, and the uncertainty and fear that accompany it, require Herculean efforts on the part of parents if their babies and children are to experience secure attachment (Moeller et al., 2013:17). Bronfenbrenner (1974) suggested that the best way of ensuring that all children achieve their potential is to provide the families of the most disadvantaged children with an adequate income, a good diet, decent housing and ready access to healthcare.

Ultimately, therefore, the state must take responsibility for creating the optimum conditions for positive parenting. Policy must play its part in reducing the risk factors that lead to poor early parenting and that nourish the relentless cycle of disadvantage, low aspirations and human misery (Moeller et al., 2013:20). Early parenting education has a role, but it is not the whole story.

Key points

Aims of early parenting education

- To increase self-efficacy for labour and birth
- To improve sensitivity to infants
- To enhance practical parenting skills
- To reduce parental stress and support mental health
- To strengthen the couple relationship across the transition to parenthood
- To build social support
- To build strong, healthy communities
- To ameliorate social inequalities

References

Braveman, P., Acker, J., Arkin, E., Bussel, J., Wehr, K. et al. (2018) *Early Childhood is Critical to Health Equity*. Robert Wood Johnson Foundation. Available at: www.rwjf.org/en/library/research/2018/05/early-childhood-is-critical-to-health-equity.html?cid=xtw_rwjf_unpd_dte:20180612 (accessed 26 October 2018).

Bronfenbrenner, U. (1974) *A Report on Longitudinal Evaluations of Preschool Programs, Volume II: Is Early Intervention Effective?* Washington, DC: US Department of Health, Educational Welfare and the National Institute of Education.

Brooks-Gunn, J., Leventhal, T., Duncan, G.J. (2000) Why poverty matters for young children: Implications for policy. In: Osofsky, J.D., Fitzgerald, H.E. (Eds.) *WAIMH Handbook of Infant Mental Health (Vol. 3): Parenting and Child Care*. New York: John Wiley, pp.89-131.

Burton-White, L. (1978) *The First Three Years of Life*. London: W.H. Allen.

Care Quality Commission (2015) *Survey of Women's Experiences of Maternity Care*. London: Care Quality Commission.

Domoney, J., Iles, J., Ramchandani, P. (2013) Paternal depression in the postnatal period: Reflections on current knowledge and practice. *International Journal of Birth and Parent Education*, 1(3):17-20.

Donkin, A., Roberts, J., Tedstone, A., Marmot, M. (2014) Family socio-economic status and young children's outcomes. *Journal of Children's Services*, 9(2):83-95.

Doss, B.D., Rhoades, G.K., Stanley, S.M., Markman, H.J. (2009) The effect of the transition to parenthood on relationship quality: An 8-year prospective study. *Journal of Personality and Social Psychology*, 96:601–609.

Early Intervention Foundation (2019) Reducing parental conflict hub. Available at: https://reducingparentalconflict.eif.org.uk/about/hub.html (accessed 8 April 2019).

Feinberg, M.E., Kan, M.L. (2008) Establishing Family Foundations: Intervention effects on coparenting, parent/infant well-being, and parent–child relations. *Journal of Family Psychology*, 22(2):253–263.

Gagnon, A.J., Sandall, J. (2007) Individual or group antenatal education for childbirth or parenthood, or both. *Cochrane Database of Systematic Reviews*, Issue 3. Art. No.: CD002869.

Gilmer, C., Buchan, J.L., Letourneau, N., Bennett, C.T., Shanker, S.G. et al. (2016) Parent education interventions designed to support the transition to parenthood: A realist review. *International Journal of Nursing Studies*, 59:118–133.

Glade, A.C., Bean, R.A., Vira, R. (2005) A prime time for marital/relational intervention: A review of the transition to parenthood literature with treatment recommendations. *The American Journal of Family Therapy*, 33(4):319–336.

Gutman, L.M., Feinstein, L. (2010) Parenting behaviours and children's development from infancy to early childhood: Changes, continuities and contributions. *Early Child Development and Care*, 180(4):535–556.

Gutman, L., Brown, J., Akerman, R. (2009) *Nurturing Parenting Capability: The Early Years*. Report No. 30. London: Centre for Research on the Wider Benefits of Learning Research.

Hanna, B.A., Edgecombe, G., Jackson, C.A., Newman, S. (2002) The importance of first-time parent groups for new parents. *Nursing and Health Science*, 4:209–214.

Howard, K.S., Brooks-Gunn, J. (2009) Relationship supportiveness during the transition to parenting among marred and unmarried parents. *Parenting, Science and Practice*, 9:123–142.

Kassebaum, N.J., Bertozzi-Villa, A., Coggeshall, M.S., Shackelford, K.A., Steiner, C. et al. (2014) Global, regional, and national levels and causes of maternal mortality during 1990–2013: A systematic analysis for the Global Burden of Disease Study 2013. *The Lancet*, 384(9947):980–1004.

Kiernan, K.E., Mensah, F.K. (2011) Poverty, family resources and children's early educational attainment: The mediating role of parenting. *British Educational Research Journal*, 37(2):317–336.

Lieberman, A.F., Van Horn, P. (2013) Infants and young children in military families: A conceptual model for intervention. *Clinical Child and Family Psychological Review*, 16:282–293.

Maternal Mental Health Alliance (2014) *Costing Perinatal Mental Health and Understanding Cost-effectiveness*. London: Maternal Mental Health Alliance.

McVeigh, C.A. (2000) Satisfaction with social support and functional status after childbirth. *Maternal and Child Nursing*, 25(1):25–30.

Mitchell, R.E., Billings, A.G., Moos, R.H. (1982) Social support and well-being: Implications for prevention programs. *Journal of Primary Prevention*, 3(2):77–98.

Moeller, M.P., Carr, G., Seaver, L., Stredler-Brown, A., Holzinger, D. (2013) Best practices in family-centered early intervention for children who are deaf or hard of hearing: An international consensus statement. *Journal of Deaf Studies and Deaf Education*, 18(4):429–445.

Molinuevo, D. (2013) *Parenting Support in Europe*. Dublin: European Foundation for the Improvement of Living and Working Conditions.

NHS Digital (2017) Maternity Services Monthly Statistics – May 2017. Available at: https://digital.nhs.uk/data-and-information/publications/statistical/maternity-services-monthly-statistics/may-2017 (accessed 29 January 2019).

O'Mahoney, F., Hofmeyr, G.J., Menon, V. (2010) Choice of instruments for assisted vaginal delivery. *Cochrane Systematic Review*. Available at: www.cochranelibrary.com/cdsr/doi/10.1002/14651858.CD005455.pub2/abstract (accessed 29 January 2019).

Parliamentary Office of Science and Technology (POST) (2002) *Caesarean Sections*. London: POST.

Public Health England (2014) *Good Quality Parenting Programmes*. London: PHE Publications.

Schlossman, S.L. (1976) Before Home Start: Notes toward a history of parent education in America, 1897-1929. *Harvard Educational Review*, 46(3):436-467.

Scott, D., Brady, S., Glynn, P. (2001) New mother groups as a social network intervention: Consumer and maternal and child health nurse perspectives. *Australian Journal of Advanced Nursing*, 18(4):23-29.

Scottish Coalition supporting Putting the Baby IN the Bath Water (2014) *Social Justice Begins with Babies*. Available at: www.bacaph.org.uk/blog/59-blog-item1-18 (accessed 23 November 2019).

Sher, J. (2016) *Missed Periods: A Primer on Preconception Health, Education and Care*. An independent report commissioned by NHS Greater Glasgow and Clyde (Public Health). Available at: www.drugsandalcohol.ie/26068/1/missed-periods-Scotand_pregnancies.pdf (accessed 23 November 2019).

Smith, D., Smith, H.L. (1978) Toward improvements in parenting: A description of prenatal and postpartum classes with teaching guide. *Journal of Obstetric and Gynecological Nursing*, November/December:22-27.

Smith, H., Peterson, N., Lagrew, D., Main, E. (2016) *Toolkit to Support Vaginal Birth and Reduce Primary Cesareans: A Quality Improvement Toolkit*. Stanford, CA: California Maternal Quality Care Collaborative.

The Scottish Government (2012a) *Bringing Up Children: Your Views*. Edinburgh: The Scottish Government.

The Scottish Government (2012b) *National Parenting Strategy: Making a Positive Difference to Children and Young People Through Parenting*. Edinburgh: The Scottish Government.

Verbiest, S., Malin, C.K., Drummonds, M., Kotelchuck, M. (2016) Catalyzing a reproductive health and social justice movement. *Maternal and Child Health Journal*, 20:741-748.

Vimpani, G. (2001) The role of social cohesiveness in promoting optimum child development. *Youth Suicide Prevention Bulletin*, 5:20-24.

Waliski, A., Bokony, P., Kirchner, J.E. (2012) Combat-related parental deployment: Identifying the impact on families with pre-school age children. *Journal of Human Behavior in the Social Environment*, 22(6):653-670.

WAVE Trust (2013) *Conception to Age 2: The Age of Opportunity*. Croydon: WAVE Trust.

Wharton, K.R., Ecker, J.L., Wax, J.R. (2017) Approaches to limit intervention during labor and birth – Committee on Obstetric Practice. *Obstetrics and Gynecology*, 129(2):e20-e28.

3   Effective parent educators
Skills and relationships

To work effectively with parents, programme staff have to be prepared, skilled and have a clear idea of the boundaries of their role.

(Molinuevo 2013:37)

The transition to parenthood presents a *uniquely valuable opportunity* to offer all new families preventative education and support, and extra interventions to families most in need. Educators therefore need to prepare for this responsibility by enhancing their understanding of the critical 1000 days, and developing the skills required to enable them to provide effective, responsive early parenting education.

Training of educators

There are few things that annoy teachers more in any area of education than the popular myth that 'those who can, do, and those who can't, teach'. Yet, inside the healthcare professions, it appears to have been believed for decades that professionals are equipped to offer education either to individuals or in groups simply by virtue of their having a clinical qualification. The skills of diagnosis, of treatment and care may have some overlap with those of education, but educators require many other skills not required by the clinician (and vice versa). The United Nations has stated:

Governments are recommended to provide .... professional training in posi-tive parenting.

(United Nations 2008)

In a review of parenting education and support across Europe, Molinuevo (2013:4) concludes that, 'the effective delivery of parenting education services requires a workforce with adequate skills' and commends those countries where this is taken seriously:

> *In Austria, parent support practitioners are required to undergo a 500 hour training programme that is focused on parenting education.*
>
> (Molinuevo 2013:2)

The link between training and education of professionals, and the effectiveness of early parenting education, has been made by Pinquart and Teubert (2010), who note that the impact of parenting education is dependent upon a variety of factors, including the qualification of the intervener and the delivery mode. Professionals need to have initial preparation for their role as early parent educators and ongoing education to ensure that they maintain the highest standards of practice (Moeller et al., 2013:430). Similarly, those in the voluntary sector providing education across the transition to parenthood – and it is considered by Sher (2016b) that the voluntary sector *should* be involved in parenting education – must also undertake training and have access to continuing professional development and assessment overseen by internal and external moderators to ensure the quality, relevance and freedom from bias of the programmes being offered to families.

Role of the educator

Successful groups, where learning in the cognitive, physical, emotional and social domain occurs, are those which are facilitated so as to create an environment of trust and a sense of group cohesion (Hanna et al., 2002). It might be argued that the era of perinatal education where parents meet in person is past and that online education, and indeed online peer support, is an adequate (if not better) substitute for 'real-world' groups. While offering parenting education via the internet might be attractive to commissioners concerned with saving money, it does not meet parents' preferences and needs. The Scottish Government's *National Parenting Strategy* (2012b) reported that, 'face to face is better than any leaflet or website' and that:

> *Parents want personal, empathetic support from individuals; technological resources are seen as supplemental to individualised information and two-way communication.*
>
> (The Scottish Government 2012b:xi)

The Dad Project (Hogg, 2014) has noted that online sources of information are not necessarily trusted by fathers and partners; talking to professionals, and even hard-copy information, is preferred to the internet. Smith (2014) stresses that we cannot attempt to help a woman build a relationship with her unborn baby if we do not first build a relationship with her. Women's satisfaction or dissatisfaction with maternity care has historically been immediately related to the quality of their interpersonal relationships with health professionals (Davis, 2013).

The role of professionals in delivering early parenting education has changed radically over the last 50 years. In her globally famous *A Textbook for Midwives*, Margaret Myles stated in the 1968 edition that women are to be 'instructed', 'advised' and 'persuaded' (to do as they are told by their midwife). The pregnant woman is seen as highly dependent, firstly on her midwife for everything from her clinical care to advice on the day-to-day running of her life, and secondly on her husband 'who determines her mood and her beauty' (Myles, 1971:724)! Not so in the 21st century when the role of professionals:

> *is increasingly conceptualised as largely one of facilitation – preparing, supporting and assisting parents to act effectively as their child's first and primary educators, protectors and health promoters...to enhance capacity and competence in early parenting.*

> (The Scottish Government 2012a:3)

The attributes of the contemporary parent educator are not those of the autocrat or even the expert; what is required is empathy, honesty, respect, humour, enthusiasm, flexibility and warmth (Hanna et al., 2002) to enable them to walk alongside new parents, rather than in front of them. A didactic approach is unhelpful and ineffective when parents need to find solutions to both the universal challenges that have confronted parents down the ages, and also to the unique challenges of their individual circumstances. There is still a place for information giving as well as sharing, but information will not change behaviour unless parents have had the opportunity to discuss it and reflect on how it can be applied in their own real-world situations. Educators must recognise that families need support inside 'their typical lives' (Moeller et al., 2013:432) and that 'decision-making authority rests with the family' (Moeller et al., 2013:434). Therefore, the role of the educator is to enter into a collaboration with the family to support and develop their capacity to exercise this authority. Early parenting education that truly embodies the principles of adult education, and educates for enhanced autonomy, does not suggest to parents that there are 'experts' who know better than they do how to care for babies and bring up their small children. This simply creates dependency on professionals and undermines what Bronfenbrenner (1974:32) describes as 'the principal system (that is, the family) that not only stimulates the child's development but can sustain it through the period of childhood and adolescence'. There are no pat answers to situations that parents encounter when raising their child and any advice and guidelines must, by definition, be adapted to a variety of situations.

Educators must recognise that families need support inside their typical lives and that decision-making authority rests with the family.

Educators need to avoid imposing a normative view of 'good' parenting, based on their own ideals and upbringing. To achieve this requires them to have created the opportunity, or taken it if offered, to reflect on their own experiences of being parented and the attitudes that they have internalised about parenting. Only by understanding one's innate prejudices is it possible to maintain an openness to different views of what constitutes good parenting. Parenting is culturally specific and imposing white middle-class values or any other set of values on families from different cultures is obviously inappropriate and harmful. Instead, it is important to try to build bridges between the mother's or couple's culture and the majority one in which they are living, acknowledging the richness of both.

Parents may have very different ideas about the resources they are going to use to guide their parenting. American parents may say they will turn to websites, books, friends and professionals for advice, whereas women from India may say they will turn to their mothers-in-law. Where mothers and fathers from a Western culture may believe that 'the latest' parenting strategies are the best, others may consider that the best guidance is to be found in the wisdom of grandmothers and great-grandmothers. The degree of 'protection' that parents should provide for their young children may be viewed very differently by parents from different countries. In Norway, childhood is strongly institutionalised and most children enter state-sponsored daycare at one year. In Japan, pre-school-aged children may be allowed to run errands unsupervised by parents. Parents in Israel want to encourage self-reliance, resourcefulness and resilience in their young children and, as in Japan and Norway, strive to cultivate independence in their children from an early age. By contrast, in parts of Asia, many children co-sleep with a family member until late childhood. American and Asian parents may be very focused on their children being 'successful' and want to start grooming them for a competitive employment market from babyhood. In the Netherlands, on the other hand, parents are averse to 'pushing' their children and may be strongly opposed to their being able to read before they go to school because they feel this will separate them from their peers and negatively affect their friendships.

The educator her/himself needs to believe and encourage parents to understand that there are many different ways of raising happy children and that diversity of parenting practices is liberating. Early parenting education groups are most useful when they foster understanding that there is no single, 'correct' way to parent and that it is acceptable (and inevitable) that parents will experiment, make 'mistakes', change course and try different ways of nurturing their baby.

Early parenting education fosters understanding that there is no 'correct' way to parent; parents are encouraged to experiment and try different ways of caring for their baby.

A strengths-based approach

All contemporary, evidence-based parenting education programmes consider a strengths-based approach beneficial. Such an approach avoids parent blaming. Health and social care professionals and institutions have a long history of blaming women for adverse outcomes in their children (McIntosh, 2012). However, it is, as Sher (2016a) points out, both unkind and pointless to blame women and parents for their choices as these choices are made in the context of larger political and societal forces, and are constrained by whether they have access to such things as adequate housing, decent schools, employment, green spaces and social facilities. The conditions under which women and men make decisions about how to lead a healthy pregnancy and plan for the future of their children vary and some parents have no experience of being allowed or helped to make informed choices in their lives (Sher, 2016a). Educators also need to recognise - frustrating though this may be - that the choices parents make are not made for all time; their decision making, like everyone else's, is a continuous process:

> *Families may adapt or change decisions in response to the child's and family's changing abilities, needs, progress and emotional wellbeing.*
>
> (Moeller et al. 2013:434)

An example of this, with which every educator will be familiar, is parents' decision about how to feed their baby. Before or during pregnancy, they may decide that their baby will be breastfed but may change their minds following the birth, especially in circumstances where there is a lack of professional and peer support to carry the family through the first often challenging weeks. Rollins et al. (2016) remind us that success in breastfeeding is *not* the sole responsibility of the woman. It is, rather, a collective, societal responsibility to promote and support it.

A strengths-based approach to parenting education goes hand in hand with a philosophy of salutogenesis. Salutogenesis informs early parenting programmes that keep family wellbeing at their heart (Lindstrom & Eriksson, 2005). It is averse to programmes that are constantly focused on 'what might go wrong' during labour, birth and early parenting - such as interventions in labour; injury to the mother and/or baby during the birth; occurrence of postnatal depression; problems with breastfeeding; sleepless nights and so forth. While these are topics that may be included in an early parenting programme, they need not be allowed to dominate. A salutogenic approach conveys confidence in parenting as a joyful, positive experience that is life enhancing and focuses on parents' and children's health and wellbeing.

The educator's approach to enabling learning in early parenting education groups will be person-centred, respecting the core conditions of empathy, congruence and unconditional positive regard (Brodley, 1986). Parents are acknowledged as trying to make the best decisions they can, according to their circumstances, for the welfare of their unborn and newborn babies. Whether the educator agrees with their decisions, or considers them misguided, she demonstrates respect for parents' agency and trust in the mother's, father's/partner's ability to become the parents they want to be (Brunton & Russell, 2008; Kim et al., 2010). The essential basis for effective parenting education is 'a two-way relationship of mutual respect and trust' (Sher, 2016a:21).

> Whether the educator agrees or not with parents' decisions, s/he demonstrates respect for their agency and trust in their ability to become the parents they want to be.

Information and understanding

What parents want from a parenting education programme is very often not what they get, and not what educators think they want. The emphasis in many sessions is on information giving in the belief that the more information parents receive, the more confident they will feel in their parenting, and the more satisfied they will be with the programme. Parents *do* want information but on their terms. In the contemporary information-rich world, making choices has not become easier, but far harder, and the need to distinguish correct information from incorrect, objective information from biased, and relevant information from irrelevant, can feel frightening. Parents are increasingly anxious about the complexity and diversity of information available about parenting. Finding information is not difficult; what parents want help with is sifting through it and analysing it so that it 'has meaning for them, their child and their circumstances' (The Scottish Government, 2012a:17). Their appetite is for information that conforms to the three 'c's of clarity, conciseness and consistency (The Scottish Government, 2012b). Parents do not want information 'dumped' on them and educators must avoid information overload (Hogg, 2014).

> Parents do not want information 'dumped' on them so it is important to avoid information overload.

Having information is not sufficient; it must be accompanied by understanding. Parents can be told about the different stages of babies' development, but such information will not support them in their parenting unless they also understand that children's development is not linear. T. Berry Brazelton, the late world-famous paediatrician, used to point out at his lectures how a surge in a child's physical skills – such as learning to walk – will generally be accompanied by regression in another area, such as a return to frequent night-time waking. Children's development is uneven, with periods of progress in the acquisition of skills followed by periods of consolidation (Gutman & Feinstein, 2008). Nor do all children advance at the same rate. The *understanding* that parents need is that each baby and child is unique and that 'milestones' are textbook terms, not real-life ones.

Therefore, the topics that have been identified as of interest to parents cannot be approached simply by giving information about them, but require discussion, sharing of experiences and reflection, thus supporting the development of a realistic, nuanced understanding. Understanding liberates parents from dependency on the 'superior knowledge' of health professionals, and supports their confidence that they are the best people to interpret their child's progress and identify when all is going well and when there are problems.

Caring for a child is no longer part of the social stock of knowledge (Mechlin, 2001). The Scottish Government (2012a) has identified four key topics that parents want to explore, whether they are the parents of babies and toddlers, or of older children. These are:

1. Feeding and diet
2. Behaviour management
3. Relationships
4. Emotional wellbeing and mental health.

They want to know about the different stages of children's development, physical and social, and how to support their healthy development, and why babies and young children behave in the way they do. Gaining knowledge, acquiring new skills for looking after their baby and developing a better understanding of the way in which they want to mother or father – all of these enable parents to have a sense of control over their transition to parenthood, and gain confidence that they will be able to manage.

Social support

In a study of mothers' motivation for joining postnatal groups, Abriola (1990) reported that only *one* of their aims was to gain *information* about babies' health and development. The women were driven far more by the desire to share their experiences of motherhood and receive emotional and practical support. They wanted to observe babies of the same age as their own, and gain reassurance that their child was making progress in line with that of other children. Very importantly, they wanted to make friends in their local area and, as Scott et al. (2001) later found, simply to get out of the house.

Hanna et al. (2002) report that women join antenatal education groups in order to build their confidence as mothers and to gain reassurance that they will be able to cope. Much of this reassurance is built on the support that they gain from their peers. Being accepted as one of a group of people making the same major life transition as themselves helps parents-to-be build their new identity as a mother or father, and to feel reassured that there are people to whom they can turn who truly understand their worries and concerns:

> *Shared attitudes and values with others provide the sense of belonging and self-worth that is an important part of the human experience.*
>
> (Abriola 1990:119)

The 'magic' of providing early parenting education in groups is that a well-facilitated, cohesive group offers multiple opportunities for *sharing*. When mothers or fathers share their concerns and experiences with a health professional at a clinic appointment, there is the opportunity for them to gain *one* (significant) person's views, but these views are necessarily shaped by that person's professional role, even if s/he has recent experience of becoming a parent. In a group of peers, parents have the opportunity to contribute to and benefit from a rich mix of ideas and experiences arising from the immediacy of the transition to parenthood that all members of the group are currently undergoing. Parents rate belonging to a peer support group highly (The Scottish Government, 2012a) and Moeller et al. (2013) consider that parent-to-parent support is critical in promoting social and emotional wellbeing for families.

In order for the experience of belonging to a group to be valuable, and for it to offer parents the support that they seek and need, groups must not be too large or too diverse. Scott et al. (2001) suggest that the ideal size of a new mothers' group, for example, is seven to eight people. An antenatal group will function well if it includes around eight couples or sixteen individuals, and even a group of this size will benefit from the educator splitting it into smaller units from time to time to ensure that everyone feels sufficiently confident to share information and ideas.

Parent-to-parent support is critical in promoting social and emotional wellbeing for families.

Continuity of educator

It is common for antenatal education programmes to be led by several educators from various backgrounds in midwifery, health visiting, nursery nursing and the early years. While it might be considered valuable to offer opportunities for parents to draw on the expertise of a variety of professionals, this is to see information giving as the primary function of early parenting education programmes.

In fact, building a group that feels safe for sharing, and that becomes a social support network, requires a *consistent* educator who gets to know the group and who is able to weave together the individual elements of the programme into a coherent, relevant educational and social experience for the particular individuals in it. The UK Social Research Unit's *Better Evidence for a Better Start* (2016) states that a key factor in facilitating change is for educators to deliver entire programmes. Continuity of carer is highly valued by women on their journey through the maternity services and has been a pillar of two major maternity reports: *Changing Childbirth* in 1993 (Department of Health) and *Better Births* in 2016 (NHS England). Continuity fosters a sense of security on the part of the woman and her family, and ensures that communication is easy and clear, with both the person delivering the service and the person receiving it understanding each other's position.

The same is true in terms of early parenting education. Women and their partners are able to develop meaningful conversations across several sessions because sessions are facilitated by the same person. The skilled facilitator who delivers an entire programme is able to ensure that every discussion develops the information and ideas that have been shared in previous sessions, and can support parents to reflect ever more deeply on their attitudes and values around parenting. Supporting couples to apply information to their own circumstances is more effective when the educator has become familiar with those circumstances, and can ask questions that are specifically relevant to couples rather than more general open-ended questions. Failure to provide the same educator across all sessions of the programme risks reducing its quality in terms of the learning that takes place, the confidence that parents gain from it and the likelihood of friendship networks forming.

> When a skilled facilitator delivers an entire programme, s/he is able to ensure that every discussion develops the information and ideas that have been shared in previous sessions.

When an educator has built a relationship of trust and liking with a group, it is easier to handle strong feelings. Outbursts of emotion can be uncomfortable for everyone, although they are not necessarily counter-productive. The educator can spot the first signs of escalating emotions – raised voices, people shifting in their seats, looking down at the floor – and aim to defuse the situation. Acknowledging and working with the emotions of the group is easier for the educator who knows the group well. Maintaining a confident, calm demeanour is important, as is being able to address parents by name and with understanding of the attitudes they have manifested in previous sessions. Describing what is happening in terms of its impact on other group members who are also well known to the educator may draw the attention of parents who are loud in their disagreement to the impact of their behaviour. The educator may suggest that the group takes a break and then speak in private to the individual or couple who are upset. The trustworthiness that s/he has demonstrated in previous sessions, along with knowledge of the couple, may help dial down strong emotions, and, if appropriate, enable individuals to accept an invitation to leave the session and make contact before the next one. The likelihood of the individual or couple returning will quite probably be linked to the respect they have for the educator, and this requires that the educator has had the chance to get to know them over a number of sessions.

Evaluation

It is difficult, if not impossible, to evaluate a parenting education programme in either the short or long term as the impact of the programme cannot be isolated from the myriad influences which are acting upon individuals in the highly sensitive period of the transition to parenthood. Nevertheless, there are indicators that can be used to assess the quality of both the delivery of the programme and the learning that has been achieved.

If the programme being delivered is manualised (either an evidence-based targeted programme such as Baby Steps or The Incredible Years, or one which has been designed by the institution for which the educator works) evaluation needs to be based on fidelity to the programme. This requires the educator to challenge her or his delivery of the programme under the following headings:

- Adherence
  Was each component of the programme delivered?

- Quality
  How well was each component delivered?

- Dose
  Was an appropriate amount of time allocated to each component?

- Engagement
  Did recipients engage with the programme?

(Social Research Unit 2016:23)

Engagement is best assessed *during* each session rather than at the end. While managing the content of the session, the educator is also noting the kinds of questions that parents are asking – is there a mix of closed and exploratory questions, that is, of questions asking simply for information and questions that probe and seek to understand the topic better? Additionally, are parents making links between what is being covered in the current session and what has been covered in previous sessions? When practical skills work is undertaken, can parents remember the skills they have learned previously, and are they able to synthesise them, for example, by using a calm breathing pattern while adopting different positions for labour, and giving and receiving massage?

The educator should also consider whether the following balances were maintained in every session of the programme:

- Between the educator talking and the group members talking
- Between people sitting in their seats and moving around
- Between work done in the whole group and work done in small groups
- Between focusing on pregnancy and birth and focusing on life with a new baby
- Between group participants determining the direction of discussion and how long to give to a topic, and the educator 'managing' the session.

In addition, educators can gain invaluable feedback by inviting another skilled educator to observe their sessions. While this may feel daunting, it is, in fact, standard practice in educational institutions today, because of its perceived value, and should be an essential part of the ongoing development of the educator and the quality assurance of any early parenting education programme.

Parents themselves are clearly a key part of the educator's evaluation strategy. Their views may be sought by asking them to complete a questionnaire after each session, or at the end of the programme, or to give their feedback online via a questionnaire mailed to them following the completion of the programme. It is important to recognise that parents' views about the effectiveness of the programme, when sought *before* their babies are born, will be shaped largely by their enjoyment of the programme; their views, when sought *after* their babies are born, are more likely to be shaped by how useful they have found the programme *in practice*. It is therefore ideal to seek their views both antenatally and postnatally, although inviting parents to complete a questionnaire in the first weeks of their babies' lives may not be very successful!

Key points

Qualities of the effective educator

- Has received dedicated training to facilitate early parenting education
- Builds a relationship with the parents in the group
- Recognises that people need support inside their 'typical lives'
- Aims to enhance the autonomy of the mother, father and family
- Avoids imposing a normative view of 'good' parenting

- Fosters understanding that there is no single, 'correct' way to parent
- Adopts a salutogenic approach based on the belief that parenting is a joyful, life-enhancing experience that supports parents' and children's health and wellbeing
- Helps parents sift through information and analyse it so that it has meaning for them, their child and their circumstances
- Provides multiple opportunities for sharing and friendship making
- Leads an entire programme, not just individual sessions

References

Abriola, D. (1990) Mothers' perceptions of a postpartum support group. *Maternal-Child Nursing Journal*, 19(2):113-134.

Brodley, B.T. (1986) *Client-centred therapy – what is it? What is it not?* Presentation at the First Annual Meeting for the Development of the Person-Centered Approach. University of Chicago, September 3-7. Available at: http://world.std.co m/~mbr2/whatscct.html (accessed 17 January 2019).

Bronfenbrenner, U. (1974) *A Report On Longitudinal Evaluations of Preschool Programs, Volume II: Is Early Intervention Effective?* Washington, DC: US Department of Health, Educational Welfare and the National Institute of Education.

Brunton, P.J., Russell, J.A. (2008) The expectant brain: Adapting for motherhood. *Nature Reviews Neuroscience*, 9:11-25.

Davis, A. (2013) *Choice, Policy and Practice in Maternity Care Since 1948*. History and Policy Papers. London: Institute of Contemporary British History, Kings College, London, and University of Cambridge.

Department of Health (DoH) (1993) *Report of the Expert Maternity Group: Changing Childbirth* (Cumberlege Report). London: HMSO.

Gutman, L.M., Feinstein, L. (2008) Parenting behaviours and children's development from infancy to early childhood: Changes, continuities and contributions. *Early Child Development and Care*, 180(4):535-556.

Hanna, B.A., Edgecombe, G., Jackson, C.A., Newman, S. (2002) The importance of first-time parent groups for new parents. *Nursing and Health Science*, 4:209-214.

Hogg, S. (2014) *The Dad Project*. London: NSPCC.

Kim, P., Leckman, J.F., Mayes, L.C., Feldman, R., Wang, X. et al. (2010) The plasticity of the human maternal brain: Longitudinal changes in brain anatomy during the early post-partum period. *Behavioral Neuroscience*, 124(5):695-700.

Lindstrom, B., Eriksson, M. (2005) Salutogenesis. *Journal of Epidemiology and Community Health*, 59:440-442.

McIntosh, T. (2012) *A Social History of Maternity and Childbirth: Key Themes in Maternity Care*. London: Routledge.

Mechlin, J. (2001) Advice to historians on advice to mothers. *Journal of Social History*, 9(1):44-62.

Moeller, M.P., Carr, G., Seaver, L., Stredler-Brown, A., Holzinger, D. (2013) Best practices in family-centered early intervention for children who are deaf or hard of hearing: An international consensus statement. *Journal of Deaf Studies and Deaf Education*, 18(4):429-445.

Molinuevo, D. (2013) *Parenting Support in Europe*. Dublin: European Foundation for the Improvement of Living and Working Conditions.

Myles, M. (1968) *A Textbook for Midwives, 6th Edition*. Edinburgh: E&S Livingstone.

Myles, M. (1971) *A Textbook for Midwives, 7th Edition*. Edinburgh: Churchill Livingstone.

NHS England (2016) *Better Births: Improving Outcomes of Maternity Services in England – A Five Year Forward View for Maternity Care.* Available at: www.england.nhs.uk/wp-content/uploads/2016/02/national-maternity-review-report.pdf (accessed 9 July 2019).

Pinquart, M., Teubert, D. (2010) Effects of parenting education with expectant and new parents: A meta-analysis. *Journal of Family Psychology*, 24(3):316–327.

Rollins, N.C., Bhandari, N., Hajeebhoy, N., Horton, S., Lutter, C.K. et al. (2016) Breastfeeding 2: Why invest, and what will it take to improve breastfeeding practices? *The Lancet*, 387:491–504.

Scott, D., Brady, S., Glynn, P. (2001) New mother groups as a social network intervention: Consumer and maternal and child health nurse perspectives. *Australian Journal of Advanced Nursing*, 18(4):23–29.

Sher, J. (2016a) *Missed Periods: A Primer on Preconception Health, Education and Care.* An independent report commissioned by NHS Greater Glasgow and Clyde (Public Health). Available at: www.drugsandalcohol.ie/26068/1/missed-periods-Scotand_pregnancies.pdf (accessed 23 November 2019).

Sher, J. (2016b) *'Doing the Right Thing' for the Next Generation of Scottish Parents.* (Blog) May 27. Available at: https://scvo.org.uk/post/2016/05/27/doing-the-rights-thing-for-next-generation-of-scottish-parents (accessed 5 February 2019).

Smith, A. (2014) Honouring the intimacy and privacy of the parents' relationship with their unborn baby. *International Journal of Birth and Parenting Education*, 2(1):7–10.

Social Research Unit (2016) *Better Evidence for a Better Start.* Dartington, UK, Social Research Unit.

The Scottish Government (2012a) *Bringing Up Children: Your Views.* Edinburgh: The Scottish Government.

The Scottish Government (2012b) *National Parenting Strategy: Making a Positive Difference to Children and Young People Through Parenting.* Edinburgh: The Scottish Government.

United Nations (2008) *Concluding Observation 42d.* UN Committee.

4 Supporting parents' prenatal relationship with their baby

The mother's emotional/cognitive relationship with the baby in pregnancy is associated with both parent-infant interaction in the postnatal period and with attachment, with more optimal ratings of the relationship in pregnancy being associated with better interaction and more secure attachment.

(Barlow 2017:6)

Research and theory

Educators can do much to help build the relationship between the pregnant woman and her unborn baby. This pregnancy relationship is crucial because it predicts and shapes the quality of early mothering during the first year of life (Benoit et al., 1997; Theran et al., 2005). The same may be true of the pregnancy relationship between fathers and their unborn babies, but there is currently little knowledge about this relationship, even though, as for mothers, it may have important implications for the father-infant relationship once the baby is born (Vreeswijk et al., 2014).

A baby who is fortunate enough to receive sensitive and responsive care from his or her primary caregivers, and who is therefore able to form strong attachment relationships, has a far brighter future ahead than the baby who is not so lucky. Attachment security is related to all aspects of the baby's development: emotional, physical, cognitive and social (Sroufe, 2005).

A key aim, therefore, of parent education during pregnancy is to assist or reinforce parents' relationship with their soon-to-be-born infant. At one level, this means education to help the mother and father/partner understand the importance of and achieve a lifestyle that enables the mother to nurture the *physical* development of the baby – discussing the significance of diet, tobacco, alcohol, prescription and non-prescription drugs, exercise, rest and recreation – but on another level, it means education that helps the mother and father to *think* about their unborn child.

Pregnancy is a time when parents-to-be prepare for life as a new family by making practical arrangements but also by preparing themselves psychologically.

They start to imagine their future life with their child, and to fantasise about what he or she will be like and the kind of relationship they will have with that child (Theran et al., 2005). Research (Barlow, 2016) has explored 'maternal representations' in pregnancy – the way in which the mother starts to define herself as a mother if this is her first pregnancy, rather than as a childless woman, and the way in which she begins to see her baby as an individual with his or her own attributes and personality. Most women have all sorts of stories to tell about their unborn baby – about when he is active and when asleep, what kind of music he likes, what noises startle him, how he reacts when other people try to feel his movements, what kinds of food the mother eats that he appears to like or not like and so on. Many have a pet name for their baby which they may (or may not) choose to share with others. On the other hand, some women seem uninterested in their unborn baby; their pregnancy is simply counted off in days and weeks; it does not seem to be a period of intense exploration of the transition to motherhood and reflection on what kind of person their baby will be. Some women express hostile feelings towards their baby, considering her 'a nuisance' or 'a pest', and longing to 'be rid' of her.

> The relationship the mother has with her unborn baby predicts the quality of the relationship she will have with her baby during the first year of life.

Fathers are also developing representations of their unborn baby, but it may be more difficult for them to build a relationship with a person whose 'reality' they have not experienced in the same way as the mother, who feels her moving in her womb with increasing intensity and frequency as the pregnancy progresses. This may make the baby less 'tangible' to fathers and so harder for them to see the baby as their son or daughter. Nonetheless, it has been found that feelings of attachment to the baby increase for first-time fathers between the first and third trimester of pregnancy (Habib & Lancaster, 2010) in the same way as for first-time mothers (van Bussel et al., 2010).

Parents who have previously lost a baby may be cautious about forming a relationship with their new baby. However well the pregnancy is going, and however many times they are reassured that everything is normal, it is inevitable that worries should persist. Heazell et al. (2019) note that one coping strategy common to parents who are pregnant after a previous pregnancy-related loss is to delay attachment to the new baby, to reduce their emotional investment in case the baby dies. These parents need support to build a relationship with *this* baby who is *not* a replacement for or a clone of the previous one, but a person in his own right, needing his mother and father to get to know him in just the same committed manner as they did for the baby they lost.

Around 95% of women have developed a sense of their baby as 'a real person' by the third trimester of pregnancy (Brandon et al., 2009). One study (Huth-Bocks et al., 2011) showed that just over half of women have normal, healthy, balanced representations of their unborn baby, with about 30% feeling disengaged from their baby, and the remaining fifth having what psychologists call 'distorted' representations of their baby. This is important because such representations tend to persist into the postnatal period (Vreeswijk et al., 2012). Women who did not have a balanced view of their unborn babies tend to be more controlling in the way they mother and more hostile to their new babies.

Why do some pregnant women develop positive representations of their unborn babies, and others not? The answer to this question is complex. A range of variables has been identified as impacting the mother's relationship with her baby (Cannella, 2005); these include the amount of support she has during her pregnancy; the quality of her relationship with the key people in her life – husband/partner, own parents, siblings, friends, work colleagues; her age, racial and ethnic background, and her self-esteem and sense of being in control of her life. In addition, the relationship with the baby will be influenced by whether he is developing healthily or not, and by the mother's (and her partner's) attitude towards childbirth – whether she approaches labour with dread or with a sense that it is a challenge she can manage. Opportunities to think quietly about her baby will be influenced by the number of children she already has to care for. The presence of two or three small children in the household will affect the time and emotional space available to think about the new baby. Her own past history is also influential – whether she was abused as a child, whether she has been in an abusive relationship as an adult, and whether the current pregnancy was planned or an 'accident'. Not surprisingly, research has found that mothers who are themselves 'securely attached', as measured by the Adult Attachment Inventory (AAI), are more likely to have a baby who becomes securely attached (Madigan et al., 2015), while mothers who are insecurely attached are more likely to have infants who are insecure.

> The mother's relationship with her unborn child is impacted by the attitudes of her husband/partner, parents, siblings, friends and work colleagues, and by her age, racial and ethnic background and self-esteem.

Into practice

Jane Barlow, Professor at Oxford, offers the following advice when working with women and their families during pregnancy:

Research findings suggest the need for practitioners to work during preg-
nancy to explore the woman's thoughts and feelings about the foetus/
unborn baby, and to support those women about whom there are concerns.
The 28-week promotional Interview, conducted as part of the Healthy Child
Programme, provides a prime opportunity to do this....

(Barlow 2016:9)

Smith (2014) stresses that educators cannot attempt to help a woman (or a man) build a relationship with the unborn baby if they themselves do not first build a relationship with the parents. It is therefore important for educators to demonstrate unconditional positive regard for the mother and father, with respect for and trust in their capacity to become the parents they desire to be, and focusing on their and their baby's wellbeing, rather than fear mongering.

There are many ways in which educators leading groups in the antenatal period can nurture a relationship between the mother and her baby and between the father and his baby. With regard to the latter, it is important to remember that a study (Vreeswijk et al., 2014) found that it is the *quality* of fathers' thoughts and feelings about their unborn baby that is more important in shaping representations of their baby than the amount of time they spend thinking about her or him. Therefore, a brief period of directed thinking in an antenatal session may be highly valuable for fathers, even if, day to day, they do not think about the baby as much as their partners whose bodies continuously register the reality of the pregnancy.

Communicating with the unborn baby

While many parents-to-be will talk quite readily to and about their unborn babies, some may feel that it's a 'silly' thing to do and pointless. They may not realise that their baby is able to hear from around 16 weeks of pregnancy and that, after birth, she will be able to recognise voices, music and sounds that she has heard regularly while in the womb. Educators can 'give permission' to parents to talk to their baby by asking such questions as:

- When do you talk to your baby? What do you tell her?
- Do you ask your baby if she's having a good day?
- Do you tell him what you're doing?
- Do you explain all the preparations you are making for his arrival?

Singing, dancing and stroking

It is an excellent idea for the educator to stress the value of *singing* to the unborn baby, as singing is an important means of promoting language devel-opment in the early years (LoRe et al., 2018) and parents who begin singing to their babies in pregnancy may be more likely to continue to do so later on. Singing is also a powerful means of tension release and emotional expression for the parents. In a fascinating study (Rozada Montemurro, 1996), it was found that mothers who had sung to their babies during pregnancy were better able to calm their newborn babies and help them fall asleep than mothers who had not. These mothers also breastfed for longer. Dancing has also been found to promote bonding (Rova & Haddow, 2017). Parents do not have to dance in public – they can dance with each other and their baby in the privacy of their home!

Educators can encourage parents to communicate with their baby through touch:

- Do you rub your tummy and talk to your baby to reassure him when something stressful has happened?'
- Do you stroke your baby during the day so that he knows you're there for him?

Asking these questions and suggesting ways of engaging with the unborn baby supports parents in building their unique relationship with their baby, and in understanding how the relationship can be grown after the baby's birth through the same means. This element of antenatal preparation may be especially important for fathers/partners who can learn strategies for being with their baby that are not dependent on feeding her, thus offering them an important role in the early postnatal period if the mother is breastfeeding.

> Singing to the unborn baby, dancing during pregnancy and stroking him or her all build the mother's and father's relationship with their baby.

Encouraging wondering

Educators can integrate a focus on reflective functioning into their sessions, to help parents appreciate that their new baby will have thoughts and feelings that underlie her behaviour. To start to build such an understanding during pregnancy makes it more likely that parents will be 'mind-minded' in their approach to their newborn baby: that is, accepting her as an individual with a mind of her own, rather than a being who functions only at the level of mundane needs that must be met in a relentless cycle of feeding, cleaning and coaxing to sleep.

Parents can be invited to *wonder* about their baby:

- What kind of personality do you think your baby has?
- Which of you do you think she's most like? Or is she like someone else in your family?

- Do you think your baby has his own routine – does he do certain things at certain times of the day?
- Do you think your baby has feelings? How do you think your baby is feeling at this moment?

Educators need to invite parents to *wonder* about their unborn baby. This encourages 'mind-mindedness': that is, parents' understanding that the baby has a mind of her own, and thoughts that underpin her behaviour.

Dreams

Educators may gain valuable insights into parents' representations of their unborn babies by asking about their dreams. While mothers and fathers-to-be who are from Western cultures may treat dreams lightly, parents from other backgrounds may consider them to be prophetic. These parents are more likely to ask themselves what their dreams mean, and to reflect on them seriously, than parents from minority countries (Maldonado-Morales, 2018). It is important, therefore, that educators are respectful of parents' dreams, and interested in them, asking the parents for their interpretations. Their answers may give considerable insight into their feelings, fears and aspirations for their baby.

Key points

Knowledge base

- The relationship the mother (and probably, the father) has with the *unborn* baby is crucial because it predicts and shapes the quality of early parenting during the first year of life
- The mother's relationship with her unborn baby is impacted by the amount of support she has, the quality of her relationship with the key people in her life, her age, racial and ethnic background, and her self-esteem and sense of being in control of her life
- Parents who are pregnant after a previous pregnancy-related loss often delay commitment to the new baby; these parents need sensitive and special support to build a relationship with their unborn child

Into practice

- Educators cannot help a mother (or a father) build a relationship with the unborn baby if they do not first build a relationship with the parents

- Educators need to work during pregnancy to explore the woman's thoughts and feelings about her unborn baby, and to support women who are finding it difficult to have a relationship with their baby
- Educators can 'give permission' to parents to talk and sing to their baby, and to dance during pregnancy, all of which promote bonding. They can also encourage parents to communicate with their baby through touching, stroking and massaging the baby in the womb
- Parents should be invited to *wonder* about their baby
- Educators need to be respectful of parents' dreams, asking parents for their interpretations as these may give insight into their feelings, fears and aspirations for their baby

References

Barlow, J. (2016) The relationship with the unborn baby: Why it matters. *International Journal of Birth and Parent Education*, 4(1):5-10.

Barlow, J. (2017) The relationship with the unborn child: Why it matters. AIMH UK Best Practice Guidance (BPG) No 4. *International Journal of Birth and Parent Education* (supplement).

Benoit, D., Parker, K.C.H., Zeanah, C.H. (1997) Mothers' representations of their infants assessed prenatally: Stability and association with infants' attachment classifications. *Journal of Child Psychology and Psychiatry*, 38(3):307-313.

Brandon, A.R., Pitts, S., Denton, W.H., Stringer, C.A., Evans, H.M. (2009) A history of the theory of prenatal attachment. *Journal of Prenatal and Perinatal Psychology and Health*, 23(4):201-222.

Cannella, B.L. (2005) Maternal-fetal attachment: An integrative review. *Journal of Advanced Nursing*, 50(1):60-68.

Habib, C., Lancaster, S. (2010) Changes in identity and paternal-foetal attachment across a first pregnancy. *Journal of Reproductive and Infant Psychology*, 28:128-142.

Heazell, A.E.P., Wojcieszek, A., Graham, N., Stephens, L. (2019) Care in pregnancies after stillbirth. *International Journal of Birth and Parent Education*, 6(2):23-28.

Huth-Bocks, A.C., Theran, S.A., Levendosky, A.A., Bogat, G.A. (2011) A social-contextual understanding of concordance and discordance between maternal prenatal representations of the infant and infant-mother attachment. *Infant Mental Health Journal*, 34(4):405-426.

LoRe, D., Ladner, P., Suskind, D. (2018) Talk, read, sing: Early language exposure as an overlooked social determinant of health. *Pediatrics*, 142(3):e20182007.

Madigan, S., Hawkins, E., Plamondon, A., Moran, G., Benoit, D. (2015) Maternal representations and infant attachment: An examination of the prototype hypothesis. *Infant Mental Health Journal*, 36:459-468.

Maldonado-Morales, M. (2018) *Culturally determined variations in perinatal care.* Presentation at World Association of Infant Mental Health conference, Rome, 29 May.

Rova, M., Haddow, S. (2017) Moving bodies. Ch. 9 in: Celebi, M. (Ed.) *Weaving the Cradle: Facilitating Groups to Promote Attunement and Bonding*. London: Jessica Kingsley Publishers: 120-131.

Rozada Montemurro, R. (1996) Singing lullabies to unborn children: Experiences in village Vilamarxant, Spain. *Pre- and Peri-natal Psychology Journal*, 11(1):9-16.

Smith, A. (2014) Honouring the intimacy and privacy of the parents' relationship with their unborn baby. *International Journal of Birth and Parent Education*, 2(1):7-10.

Sroufe, L.A. (2005) Attachment and development: A prospective, longitudinal study from birth to adulthood. *Attachment & Human Development*, 7(4):349-367.

Theran, S.A., Levendosky, A.A., Bogta, G.A., Huth-Bocks, A.C. (2005) Stability and change in mothers' internal representations of their infants over time. *Attachment & Human Development*, 7(3):253-268.

van Bussel, J.C.H., Spitz, B., Demyttenaere, K. (2010) Reliability and validity of the Dutch version of the maternal antenatal attachment scale. *Archives of Women's Mental Health*, 13:267-277.

Vreeswijk, C.M.J., Maas, J.B.M., van Bakel, H.J.A. (2012) Parental representations: A systematic review of the Working Model of the Child Interview. *Infant Mental Health Journal*, 33(3):314-328.

Vreeswijk, C.M.J., Maas, A., Rijk, C., van Bakel, H. (2014) Fathers' experiences during pregnancy: Paternal prenatal attachment and representations of the fetus. *Psychology of Men and Masculinities*, 15(2):129-137.

5 Stress and relaxation
Education for a calm pregnancy

Ancient Chinese texts speak of the importance of protecting the pregnant woman from unpleasant experiences, of ensuring that she is told uplifting stories and that she is relaxed and able to sleep peacefully at night. Vedic scriptures recommend that pregnant women should try to be happy and in a pleasant mood at all times because this will affect their unborn baby's temperament. The mother-to-be should keep an internal balance so that her baby's future will be equally well balanced.

(Nolan 2015:3)

Research and theory

In the early 20th century, advice given to the mother during pregnancy would have been largely around avoiding physical hazards, such as taking care not to trip or fall, and resting when she could. Little was known about the impact of diet on the development of the unborn baby and, by and large, women would have continued to eat what they normally ate, given that choice of diet was, in any case, a luxury reserved for the rich. What was going on in the woman's *mind* as she prepared for motherhood was known only to her – whether she was or wasn't bonding with her unborn child, what representations she had of her baby, whether she had much time to think about the baby at all.

For working women, pregnancy was often a burden on top of the other hardships which defined their lives. Childbirth was to be feared as an occasion of injury to the mother, exhaustion, possible death and, finally, as the event leading to the arrival of another mouth to feed.

Of course, for millions of women today in both developing majority and affluent minority countries, pregnancy is experienced largely as it has been for thousands of years. Pressures related to new understanding of how babies develop and what their growing brains need coming from neuroscience, developmental psychology, obstetrics and midwifery probably weigh most heavily on women generally considered to be privileged – the educated, the well-off and those who are in a position to make choices.

Understanding of the multiple links between mother and unborn child – physical, emotional and spiritual – is not, however, new. There was in early civilisations a profound appreciation of the connection between the woman and her unborn baby, and of the way in which the mind of the mother touched the baby's mind (Vincent-Priya, 1992). The Chinese have understood from ancient times that what affects a pregnant woman's state of mind will also affect the unborn baby in the womb. The mother is therefore encouraged to be calm and to surround herself with beautiful things during pregnancy. Before she goes to sleep at night, she is advised to read or have read to her uplifting stories to ensure positive imaginings in her dreams. Chinese traditional practices during pregnancy include singing, which is considered to promote calm in both mother and unborn baby, a calm which will affect the child's temperament after birth. Vedic scriptures dating back to a thousand years before Christ recommend that pregnant women should be helped to be happy and to achieve a healthy balance in all aspects of their lives so that their babies will be similarly well balanced.

Late-20th-century and early-21st-century research has merely confirmed these age-old insights. We know that the unborn baby cannot avoid the mother's world. He or she is inescapably linked to it. The baby's brain is registering experiences as early as 20 weeks of pregnancy when neurons have been observed firing in response, for example, to a vibration stimulus (Moore et al., 2011), or to music (Sallenbach, 1993) or loud noises (Reissland et al., 2013). Babies recognise their mothers' voice at birth, having long become accustomed to it during their time in the womb, and prefer music they have heard played regularly during pregnancy (Moon et al., 2012).

> Pregnancy prepares the baby to manage the world into which she is going to be born.

From the womb onwards, nature helps the baby to prepare for and manage the world into which she is going to be born. Adaptations to the functioning of major organs, and the formation of specific pathways in the brain, help ready the unborn baby for the outside world, be that a world in which food is plentiful or problematic, a world in which her mother feels safe or frightened. The baby probably 'reads' the mother's vital signs, that is her heart rate, her blood pressure and her body temperature, and then prepares at the physical and cognitive level to cope with the level of 'threat' that the vital signs suggest (DiPietro et al., 2008). If the baby is developing in the womb of a woman who has an unreliable eating pattern, perhaps taking in insufficient food, or bingeing and then purging, the baby is able to store more or less fat in order to compensate, and controls the blood flow to the brain and liver in order to achieve this (Godfrey et al., 2012).

The pregnant woman not only influences the physical development of her unborn baby by the food she eats, what she drinks, the drugs she takes, the poisons she ingests in the form of tobacco and alcohol, and the external hazards to which she is exposed such as radiation and pollution, she also influences the development of her baby's brain through stress hormones which she (involuntarily) passes across the placenta. It has been hypothesised that if a pregnant woman produces a large amount of cortisol in response to stress in her life, the placenta cannot convert all of it into an inactive form as it is able to do when cortisol is at a normal level. Glover et al. (2009) believe that cortisol in excess of the 10-20% that normally passes to the baby may be harmful. Raised levels of maternal hormones such as dopamine and serotonin which pass to the unborn baby lower the baby's and child's tolerance of stress, increase her likelihood of having problems such as attention deficit hyperactivity disorder (ADHD) (Van den Bergh & Marcoen, 2004) and adversely affect her immature immune system (Howerton & Bale, 2012).

> Raised levels of maternal dopamine and serotonin in pregnancy lower the baby's tolerance of stress, adversely affect his immature immune system and increase his likelihood of having problems such as ADHD.

Exposure of the pregnant woman, and therefore of her baby, to major traumatic events such as natural disasters, war and terrorist attacks appears to have prolonged consequences, as illustrated in an early study of the impact of 9/11 on the children of women who witnessed the destruction of the Twin Towers (Yehuda et al., 2005). The acute stress associated with such catastrophes is, however, no more serious for the unborn baby than the chronic stress her mother may be experiencing as a result of poverty, living in a situation of domestic abuse or having poor mental health. Research has shown that babies manage stimuli differently according to their mother's state of mental health. If a pregnant woman is suffering from depression, her unborn baby's heart rate increases to a higher rate in response to a stressful stimulus and takes longer to return to its normal baseline than the heart rate of a baby whose mother is enjoying good mental health (Dieter et al., 2001).

If a mother is stressed when pregnant, it also appears that her baby is more likely to be born early and to be small for dates (Wadhwa et al., 1993). Being born prematurely is disadvantageous as the brain develops until term at 40 weeks and babies born well before this, or even a little, miss out on this final phase of development (Kugelman & Colin, 2013). Low birthweight is predictive of ill health extending into adulthood (Barker et al., 2001) and the stress the baby has experienced vicariously in the womb makes her more vulnerable to emotional, cognitive and physical problems during childhood (Talge et al., 2007).

The baby's, child's and adult's stress thermometer seems to be calibrated in the womb. Unborn babies who are exposed to a high emotional temperature may experience the consequences throughout their lives, including negative impacts on their capacity to regulate their emotions and behaviour, and on their ability to learn and apply knowledge and skills (Pesonen et al., 2013). However, research is not as yet able to throw light on whether it is the *timing* of stressful events in pregnancy, the *severity* of stress or the *continuity* of stress that has the greatest impact on the unborn baby. For example, it might be that the ongoing confusion and anxiety experienced by a migrant woman may have a greater impact on her unborn child owing to its being the condition of her day-to-day life than the acute terror, followed by restoration of normal levels of stress, experienced by a woman caught up in a hurricane. The mother transfers her own experience of the world she is in to her baby, but research cannot yet tell us whether a world of ongoing stress, or one in which the mother experiences a sudden surge of stress quickly resolved, is the more harmful to the unborn baby.

It is therefore important for educators to understand that research into the impact of maternal stress in pregnancy on the baby's developing brain is in its infancy. Already there are dissenting voices which are challenging whether *all* unborn babies experience stress in utero in the same way. Jay Belsky (2018), eminent American child psychologist, argues that unborn babies and children are not *equally* susceptible to maternal stress. He considers that some babies may be shaped by their developmental experiences, both intra-uterine and extra-uterine, more than others. He talks about a 'gradient of susceptibility' and argues that nurture may be a more powerful influence on some individuals than nature, while for others, nature is more powerful.

> Research into the impact of maternal stress during pregnancy is in its infancy. It is not known whether it is the *timing* of stressful events, the *severity* of stress or *continuity* of stress that has the greatest impact on the unborn baby.

As the research stands at present, it is not possible to predict which unborn babies will be most affected by maternal stress, and which less so or possibly, not at all. It could be that too little stress in utero is not good for babies either, as there is some evidence that children's cognitive abilities are enhanced if their mothers were stressed in pregnancy (Karlsson, 2018). Overall, it is safe to assume that the best means of safeguarding the healthy development of the unborn and newborn baby's brain is to look after the pregnant and new mother. Therefore, it is a logical and compassionate way forward to educate *all* mothers about the benefits of reducing stress in pregnancy, and to help each one to find her own strategies for coping with stress. Such strategies are life skills that she can draw on across the transition to parenthood and long after pregnancy is over.

Into practice

Education in pregnancy is an opportunity for mothers to acquire relaxation skills which will help them provide a calm intra-uterine environment for their unborn baby, manage the intensity of contractions during labour and cope with the stresses of new parenthood. A systematic review of the literature on relaxation in pregnancy (Fink et al., 2012) concluded that pregnant women who practise relaxation have fewer preterm babies, fewer obstetric complications and are less likely to require a caesarean section. Which relaxation techniques are more helpful in calming anxiety in pregnancy has been explored by Urech et al. (2010). These researchers found that different types of relaxation target different psychological and biological stress systems. Guided imagery appears to induce a deep state of relaxation, but progressive muscular relaxation is equally effective in slowing the heart rate. Relaxation training is now central to several evidence-based parent education programmes, such as Baby Steps, Mellow Bumps, Hypnobirthing and Mindfulness-Based Birth and Parent Education.

The environment for relaxation

If including relaxation practice in early parenting education sessions is to be effective in achieving a calm intra-uterine environment for the baby, it must be valued by the educator as an integral part of the programme and given sufficient time in each session for skills to become well established and for parents to become confident in using them.

Smith (2014) makes the following key points about teaching relaxation:

> The emotional and physical environment in the room where relaxation strategies are to be tried out (the 'nest') should be carefully prepared with consideration given to warmth, privacy, comfort, lighting, quiet and gentle music. (p9)

It is clearly helpful if the room in which relaxation sessions take place is safe from interruptions and offers participants a choice of chairs, bean bags, pillows and mattresses to make themselves comfortable. Dim lighting and gentle music are also helpful. However, even in a less than ideal environment, an educator who understands how her/his own body reacts when stressed and is thoroughly acquainted with the impact of relaxation in her/his own life (Nolan, 2015) will be able to provide a positive experience of relaxation for mothers and fathers.

Educators cannot successfully convey the benefits of relaxation if they are obviously not relaxed themselves. Rushing into a parent education session at the last minute, and being disorganised and flustered, sends out messages that undermine what she or he is trying to convey about the importance of relaxation. Common sense suggests that if educators are tense, worrying about the content of the session they are leading, or the work they have to do during the rest of the day, or are pressed for time, they will transmit tension to the parents attending the session.

> To be truly congruent, the educator should be familiar with using relaxation strategies, positive affirmations and visualisation to good effect in her/his own life.

Introducing relaxation

Smith (2014) suggests that 'doing relaxation' may be uncomfortable for some mothers and fathers, or totally unfamiliar to them. Relaxation strategies can be made to feel less intimidating if presented simply as opportunities to add to parents' pre-existing repertoire of skills for managing stress in their lives. All parents will be able to share ways in which they wind down; some will enjoy listening to music, walking their dog, having a long bath, cycling, cooking or just sitting quietly by a window looking out. All of these are opportunities while pregnant for thinking about the baby and life as a parent. Parents can also identify what effect relaxation has on their bodily systems: they know that their muscles feel less tense when they are relaxed; headaches disappear; hands and feet are warmer or less sweaty; digestion is better; movement is more fluid and speech comes more easily. They are familiar with the fact that blood pressure drops and heart rate slows when the body moves from a stressed to a non-stressed state.

Guided relaxation sessions can be built on this basis of everyday experience and understanding. If the parenting education programme is running across several weeks, the educator has the opportunity to offer participants a variety of relaxation techniques so that each individual can identify which suits him or her best. Alongside leading longer sessions during which participants can enter into a deeply relaxed state and visualise their baby and their future together, the educator can also introduce quick relaxation techniques for dealing in the moment with stressful situations. Mothers and fathers will readily identify everyday stresses, such as being late for an antenatal appointment; feeling overwhelmed by having too much to do; joining a long queue at the check-out when they're in a hurry; coping with a puppy who's had 'an accident'; being the butt of a sharp rejoinder or thoughtless comment from a colleague or family member. For such situations, the calm breathing techniques which form the introduction to and the basis of relaxation can be quickly applied: a deep breath in and a long, slow, sighing out-breath; another in-breath followed by a longer out-breath while dropping the shoulders and loosening the jaw. The mantra for parents to take away is *sigh out slowly* (SOS), focusing on releasing tension on the out-breath. As an introduction to the power of relaxation, it is a simple strategy and transparent in its mode of working and in its effectiveness.

> Concentrating for a couple of seconds on breathing 'in' and 'out', dropping the shoulders and letting go of tension on the out-breath, is an effective strategy for tackling stress-laden situations.

Group participants need to work with their *own* breathing pattern. Some people naturally breathe deeply, others more shallowly with shorter in-breaths and out-breaths. While deep breathing that reaches the lower segments of the lungs might, physiologically, be considered optimum, not everyone can breathe in this way. The educator's task is to raise each individual's awareness of her or his own breathing pattern, and of how their in-breath and their out-breath are rhythmical and balanced. An invitation to slightly lengthen the out-breath can lead to slower, calmer breathing. Some people will respond comfortably to an instruction to breathe in for a count of five and out for a count of six, for example, but others will find themselves having to force their natural breathing pattern. Instead, participants might be invited to concentrate on their breathing, and then to say to themselves '*in*' as they breathe in and '*out*' as they breathe out, making sure to sound the 't' of 'out'. Silently sounding the 't' will increase the length of the out-breath, which is the breath on which stress is released both physically and psychologically.

Helping participants feel safe in undertaking a relaxation session is vital. Being asked to close their eyes might feel very threatening to some individuals. Participants can be invited to shut their eyes if they feel this would be helpful, or, if they prefer, to look down towards the floor and let their eyes shut when it feels natural. The educator needs to make it clear that she will also close her eyes so that group members do not need to worry that she is checking that they are following instructions 'correctly'.

Guided relaxation

Progressive muscular relaxation is a helpful exercise in demonstrating the power of relaxation. The contrast between tense muscles and relaxed ones is made very evident. A typical script might be as follows:

Shut your eyes if you want to. If you don't, that's fine. If your eyes start to feel heavy, let them gently close when you are ready.

Become aware of your own breathing. The in-breath and the out-breath. Your breathing is rhythmical. If your attention wanders away from your breathing, bring it gently back to your in-breath and your out-breath.

Now every time you breathe out, imagine that your breath is carrying away all your tension.

Think about your legs. Press your feet firmly into the ground so that you feel the tension right the way up your calves and into your thighs. Now, as you breathe out, release that tension; let your legs feel heavy and your thighs roll slightly apart.

Think about your tummy. Pull your tummy in towards your spine. Now, as you breathe out, let your tummy muscles loosen. There's no need to hold your tummy in tightly.

Think about your hands and arms. Make a fist of your hands, Then, as you breathe out, let your fingers become gently curled; even your thumbs become slightly curved. Let your elbows rest against your body.

Think about your shoulders. So much tension can accumulate in your shoulders. Hunch them up towards your ears. As you breathe out, let your shoulders sink downwards, so that they feel loose and easy.

And finally, think about your face. You have lots of muscles that work your face. Screw your face up (remember, no one is looking at you). Now, as you breathe out, let the muscles of your face loosen and the expression on your face slip away so that your forehead is smooth, your jaw slack and your mouth perhaps slightly open.

A guided relaxation will, according to Smith (2014), have four stages:

1. A period in which the relaxed state is induced
2. Deepening the relaxed state
3. Using the relaxed state to offer positive suggestions
4. Gently bringing back out of the relaxed state. (p9)

The following is a script that follows these stages. Note that the baby is sometimes described as male and sometimes as female and that the script aims to be inclusive of both mother and father, avoiding language that includes only the mother, such as 'your womb' and 'the baby inside you'.

Focus on your breathing. Notice how rhythmical your in-breath and your out-breath are. Your breathing is one of the essential rhythms of life. Sink into your breathing, letting each out-breath carry away all your tension.

Spend a moment appreciating how your body feels when it is truly at ease. If any part of your body feels tense, use your out-breath to cleanse the tension, letting the tension slip away as you breathe out.

Now you have time to think about your unborn baby. Your baby is warm inside the womb. He or she is hearing sounds which have become very familiar – mother's heart beat; mother's and father's voices – perhaps the voices of other family members as well; the sound of blood flowing through the placenta.

Your baby is cuddled by the walls of the womb – when he stretches out his arms, he feels the soft contours of his mother's body. When he is born, he will be surprised by the space around him and will be soothed by being held close to you.

Your baby is fed on demand while she is inside the womb. Her food is brought to her and all her waste products are taken effortlessly away. She will be in a strange new world when she's born and has to ask for food and tell you when she is uncomfortable. Feeding her and changing her will soothe her.

Your baby is uniquely your special child. He knows you and has a relationship with you that no one else can have in quite the same way.

When he is born, he will be content when you offer him the warmth and the holding that he has experienced in the womb, and when he hears the sounds that he has become familiar with. So hold him close to your heart, talk to him and keep him close to you.

Enjoy a few moments with your baby ...

Now become aware once more of your breathing: the in-breath and the long out-breath. Count through three cycles of your breathing and then open your eyes and come back into the room.

Visualisation is frequently employed to deepen the relaxed state. However, no single visualisation will appeal to everyone. Images of the sea and of the ebb and flow of waves are commonly used in relaxation sessions. It is also common for educators to evoke scenes of the countryside or of familiar rooms at home. All of these are potentially disturbing images for those frightened of water, who suffer from hay fever or who don't feel safe at home. It is therefore safer to invite parents to imagine for themselves a place or situation in which they feel relaxed.

Suggestions made during a relaxation session need to be relevant to the individuals in the group. Therefore, it is important to know something about the mothers and fathers/partners and what they are looking forward to doing with their babies. A discussion prior to practising relaxation might highlight how participants are eagerly anticipating cuddling their baby, or dressing him, or taking her out in a sling, or playing with her or singing and reading to him. These aspirations can then be included in the narrative spoken by the educator and become the focus of visualisations during the deepest moments of the relaxation activity.

If group members want a relaxation script to help them practise at home, it is not difficult to point them in the direction of resources on the internet. It makes sense for the educator to have listened to any scripts she recommends before recommending them to parents just in case they contain language or ideas that are unhelpful, inappropriate or culturally insensitive or irrelevant.

Poetry can provide a powerful stimulus for relaxation and visualisation. The following is a poem that could be read out by the educator once parents are in a relaxed state, or printed for them to take home and read to themselves during a quiet moment.

> *In utero*
> *As I grow here in the womb, I am comfortable*
> *In anticipation of our first meeting.*
>
> *I want you to know you are the most important thing*
> *In my life.*
> *I have no desire to be dressed in designer clothes,*
> *Sleep in the most innovative cot,*
> *Travel in the most expensive pram.*
> *I am only interested in you.*
>
> *I am hopeful our first meeting will be gentle.*
> *Yours is the voice I want to hear welcome me.*
> *Your hands are the hands I want to caress me.*
> *You are my safe place.*
>
> *Let us fall in love all over again.*
> *Please know that when you feed me,*
> *You are nourishing my body and my soul.*
> *You have everything I need.*
>
> *I want you to know I will be scared when you are not near me.*
> *I want you to know I have so many new sensations,*
> *Bright lights, loud noises, new tastes, cold surfaces.*
> *I need you with me, talking me through it.*
>
> *I want you to know sometimes I will cry because it is all too much*
> *And you might not know how to help me*
> *But please try, please stay with me, please talk to me,*

Please cuddle me.
Those are the things I will need,
Not toys to stimulate me, not enforced routines to encourage self-soothing,
Not a pacifier to space my feeds.

I want you to know that sometimes you will cry too,
And sometimes you won't know why.
I won't judge you for that. I love you mistakes and all.

I want you to know science is on our side.
The experts believe that love and nurture are what I need
And this is what I want you to know.

(Palin 2018 – slightly abridged)

Key points

Research and theory

- During pregnancy, adaptations to the functioning of major organs, and the formation of specific pathways in the brain, help prepare the unborn baby for the outside world
- The baby's, child's and adult's stress thermometer appears to be calibrated in the womb. Exposure to high levels of stress may impact negatively on future capacity to self-regulate, learn and apply knowledge and skills
- As yet, it is not known whether it is the *timing* of stressful events in pregnancy, or the *severity* of stress or whether it is *continuity* of stress that has the greatest impact on the unborn baby
- It may be that pregnancy stress is not experienced by all unborn babies in the same way; there may be a 'gradient of susceptibility'
- Women who practise relaxation have better pregnancy outcomes, fewer preterm babies, fewer obstetric complications and are less likely to require a caesarean section

Into practice

- The best means of safeguarding the healthy development of the unborn and newborn baby's brain is to look after the pregnant and new mother and educate *all* mothers about the benefits of reducing stress in pregnancy
- Educators cannot successfully convey the benefits of relaxation if they do not incorporate relaxation strategies into their own lives

- Relaxation skills need to be central to early parenting education programmes and given sufficient time in each session for parents to become confident in using them
- Practising relaxation strategies is less intimidating for parents if presented simply as adding to their existing repertoire of skills for managing stress in their lives
- Relaxation scripts need to be inclusive of both mother and father, avoiding language that excludes the father/partner

Note

In the Appendix is a teaching activity, 'Exploring mental health', which may be helpful in facilitating sessions which focus on stress and relaxation.

References

Barker, D.J.P., Forsen, T., Uutela, A., Osmond, C., Eriksson, J.G. (2001) Size at birth and resilience to effects of poor living conditions in adult life: A longitudinal study. *British Medical Journal*, 323(1273):1.

Belsky, J. (2018) *Differential susceptibility to environmental influences.* World Association of Infant Mental Health conference, Rome, May 26.

Dieter, J.N., Field, T., Hernandez-Reif, M., Jones, N.A., Lecanuet, J.P. et al. (2001) Maternal depression and increased fetal activity. *Journal of Obstetrics and Gynaecology*, 21(5):468–473.

DiPietro, J.A., Costigan, K.A., Nelson, P., Gurewitsch, E.D. (2008) Fetal responses to induced maternal relaxation during pregnancy. *Biochemical Psychiatry*, 77(1):11–19.

Fink, N.S., Urech, C., Cavelti, M., Alder, J. (2012) Relaxation during pregnancy: What are the benefits for mother, fetus, and the newborn? A systematic review of the literature. *The Journal of Perinatal and Neonatal Nursing*, 26(4):296–306.

Glover, V., Bergman, K., Sarkar, P., O'Connor, T.G. (2009) Association between maternal and amniotic fluid cortisol is moderated by maternal anxiety. *Psychoneuroendocrinology*, 34(3):430–435.

Godfrey, K.M., Haugen, G., Kiserud, T., Inskip, H.M., Cooper, C. et al. (2012) Fetal liver blood flow distribution: Role in human developmental strategy to prioritize fat deposition versus brain development. *PLoS ONE*, 7(8):e41759.

Howerton, C.L., Bale, T.L. (2012) Prenatal programing: At the intersection of maternal stress and immune activation. *Hormones and Behavior*, 62(3):237–242.

Karlsson, K. (2018) *Effects of prenatal stress on child brain development.* World Association of Infant Mental Health conference, Rome, May 28.

Kugelman, A., Colin, A.A. (2013) Late preterm infants: Near term but still in a critical developmental time period. *Pediatrics*, 132:741–751.

Moon, C., Lagercrantz, H., Kuhl, P.K. (2012) Language experienced in utero affects vowel perception after birth: A two-country study. *Acta Paediatrica*, 102(2):156–160.

Moore, A.R., Wen-Liang, Z., Jakovcevski, I., Zecevic, N., Antic, S.D. (2011) Spontaneous electrical activity in the human fetal cortex in vitro. *Journal of Neuroscience*, 31(7):853–857.

Nolan, M. (2015) Education for calm pregnancy. *International Journal of Birth and Parent Education*, 2(4):3–6.

Palin, C. (2018) In utero. *International Journal of Birth and Parent Education*, 6(1):8.

Pesonen, A.K, Eriksson, J.G., Heinonen, K., Kajantie, E., Tuovinen, S. et al. (2013) Cognitive ability and decline after early life stress exposure. *Neurobiology of Aging*, 34(6):1674-1679.

Reissland, N., Francis, B., Mason, J. (2013) Can healthy foetuses show facial expressions of 'pain' or 'distress'? *PLoS ONE*, 8(6):e65530.

Sallenbach, W.B. (1993) The intelligent prenate: Paradigms in prenatal learning and bonding. In: Blum, T.P. (Ed.) *Prenatal Perception, Learning and Bonding*. Hong Kong: Leonardo: 61-106.

Smith, A. (2014) Honouring the intimacy and privacy of the parents' relationship with their unborn baby. *International Journal of Birth and Parent Education*, 2(1):7-10.

Talge, N.M., Neal, C., Glover, V. (2007) Antenatal maternal stress and long-term effects on child neurodevelopment: How and why? *Journal of Child Psychology and Psychiatry and Allied Disciplines*, 48(3-4):245-261.

Urech, C., Fink, N.S., Hoesli, I., Wilhelm, F.H., Bitzer, J. et al. (2010) Effects of relaxation on psychobiological wellbeing during pregnancy: A randomized controlled trial. *Psychoneuroendocrinology*, 35(9):1348-1355.

Van den Bergh, B.R.H., Marcoen, A. (2004) High antenatal maternal anxiety is related to ADHD symptoms, externalizing problems, and anxiety in 8- and 9-year-olds. *Child Development*, 75(4):1085-1097.

Vincent-Priya, J. (1992) *Birth Traditions and Modern Pregnancy Care*. Dorset: Element Books.

Wadhwa, P.D., Sandman, A., Porto, M., Dunkel-Schetter, C., Garite, T.J. (1993) The association between prenatal stress and infant birth weight and gestational age at birth: A prospective investigation. *American Journal of Obstetrics and Gynecology*, 169(4):858-865.

Yehuda, R., Mulherin Engel, S., Brand, S.R., Seckl, J., Marcus, S.M. et al. (2005) Transgenerational effects of posttraumatic stress disorder in babies of mothers exposed to the World Trade Center attacks during pregnancy. *Journal of Clinical Endocrinology & Metabolism*, 90(7):4115-4118.

6 Education and support for normal birth

It is crucial that we, as childbirth educators, recognize that we do not just provide information about pregnancy and birth, but that we have the power to inspire and influence how a couple perceives birth and subsequently experiences birth. We can profoundly affect a couple's birth experience in either positive or negative ways, and hence their ongoing journey as a family.

(Jackson 2014:14)

Research and theory

The majority of women would like to have a straightforward vaginal birth with no interventions (Care Quality Commission, 2015; Wharton et al., 2017). It has long been accepted that procedures such as acceleration of labour, assisted delivery with forceps and ventouse, and surgical birth by caesarean section carry both physical and psychological risks (NCT/RCM/RCOG, 2007). Conversely, research has demonstrated that birth *without* interventions has many benefits, including reduced maternity care costs, and improved physical and psychological outcomes for women (O'Mahoney et al., 2010; Kassebaum et al., 2014; Smith et al., 2016). In their seminal paper on optimising caesarean section use, Betrán and colleagues (2018) conclude that 'in many settings, the current frequency of CS [caesarean section] cannot be medically justified'. They also note:

> *Contrary to perceived opinion…most women around the world do not prefer a CS in the absence of current or previous complications.*

(pp1358-9)

The educator's role is to help every woman and her chosen birth partner to experience giving birth positively, and to maximise their capacity to work with the physiological process of labour in order to reap the benefits that normal labour provides for the baby and mother. Additionally, educators have a responsibility to recalibrate the cultural scales of childbirth which have been tipping more and more in recent decades towards unquestioning faith in a medicalised, technocratic paradigm. There is little evidence that maximising the use of technology during labour and increasing medical surveillance of labouring women lead to improved outcomes (Sandall et al., 2016). As adult education aims to increase women's and men's autonomy, and their ability to make considered choices, it is important that early parenting education should enable mothers, fathers and partners to reflect on the way in which they want their babies to come into the world. In the interests of embracing a salutogenic approach to early parenting education, with an emphasis on working with people's strengths so as to achieve a positive transition to parenthood, educators have a responsibility to help parents gain a deeper understanding of the physiology of normal labour and of how women can work harmoniously with their bodies. The educator may feel she has, in any case, a moral obligation to do everything she can to support normal labour given the evidence that intervening in the labours of essentially healthy women who have had straightforward pregnancies is likely to cause more harm than good (Brownlee et al., 2017).

> Adult education aims to increase individuals' autonomy, so it is important that early parenting education should enable mothers, fathers and partners to make considered choices about the way in which they want their babies to come into the world.

There is a debate to be had as to whether antenatal preparation for labour and birth should focus *exclusively* on straightforward vaginal delivery with no mention of pharmacological forms of pain relief, assisted birth or caesarean section, or whether it should include information about these interventions. It is possible to argue both cases cogently. If birth interventions are included in antenatal sessions, does this risk 'normalising' them and giving mothers and their partners the impression that these are an essential/inevitable part of the contemporary birth package? If they are not included, does this risk depriving parents of information to enable them to make the choices that are right for them if they need or want to have interventions?

Wherever individual educators feel themselves to stand in the debate on the contemporary way of birth, they will nonetheless want to give the parents attending their sessions as much information about the normal progress of labour, and as many skills as possible to give them the best chance of having a physically and emotionally safe and satisfying birth without interventions.

While the profound impact of stress in pregnancy on the unborn baby is a recent topic of scientific and clinical interest, the ability to relax in labour in order to manage the intensity of contractions has long been understood by women and professionals. Since the advent of modern childbirth education with the publication of Dick-Read's *Childbirth Without Fear* in 1942, the ability to relax in labour has been recognised, not so much for the benefit that it might bring to the mother–baby relationship, but for its contribution to enabling women to have an easy birth, avoiding physical and psychological injury. From the 1950s onwards, the rejection by some women of the medicalisation of childbirth, and a desire for personal control, motivated them to find internal resources to manage the pain of labour, rather than turning to drugs. Teaching relaxation for labour and birth was an important role for physiotherapists and health visitors in the 1970s and 1980s. Pregnant women might spend half of each antenatal class relaxing while listening to music and a script read out by the educator.

From the 1990s, with the increase in the caesarean section rate and the growth of a culture of fear around childbirth and its management in affluent countries, interest in self-help strategies has remained strong despite the ready availability of epidural analgesia. New approaches to relaxation in labour, such as hypnobirthing, continue to be based on the principles of understanding the body's response to stress and acquiring techniques for controlling it.

> In order to have the best chance of a physically and emotionally safe and satisfying birth without interventions, parents need *information* about the normal progress of labour, and *skills* to manage the intensity of contractions.

In recent years, a far greater understanding of the role of key hormones in labour has evolved, and especially of oxytocin. This is information that educators need to be able to share with parents. Oxytocin is the hormone that fuels contractions, ejects milk from the breasts and nurtures the relationship between the mother and father and their newborn child (Uvnäs-Moberg, 1998). It has, therefore, both short-term effects in labour, and a longer-term impact on attachment and bonding.

During labour, the level of oxytocin in the woman's body increases hugely. As the baby's head presses down on the cervix with ever greater force, it stimulates nerves that send messages to the hypothalamus via the spinal cord. Specialised areas of the hypothalamus produce oxytocin in response. Contractions become stronger as the level of oxytocin increases. In conjunction with this increase, the brain produces pain-relieving substances to mitigate the intensity of contractions for the mother. Oxytocin also has an effect on blood pressure, raising it so as to ensure that the circulation through the placenta is such as to provide maximum oxygen and nutrients for the baby during labour. The production of oxytocin is facilitated or impeded by the environment of labour; it is stimulated when a woman feels private, safe and unobserved (Buckley, 2015), and hindered when her intense inward concentration is disturbed by, for example, being asked questions and subjected to medical procedures.

Following the birth, oxytocin has a calming effect and the mother becomes focused on her baby. She feels placid. Oxytocin affects the father similarly, reducing aggression and increasing sociability. These are strategies employed by nature to protect the baby by maximising his parents' attention to his needs, and their openness to help from other adults (Uvnäs-Moberg, 2013).

Into practice

Information giving and sharing

Educators may be anxious that there is a great deal of information that needs to be given to parents in order to prepare them for the experience of labour and birth and to enable them to make informed choices about the care they want to receive. However, overloading and over-burdening parents with facts and figures is counter-productive and it is important to remember that even people with excellent memories can only retain a little new information at a time.

In order for information to be retained (and there is little point in offering it if it is *not* going to be retained), the information provided must be relevant; it must be information that parents want; it must relate to their own or other people's experiences and be presented in a variety of ways so that auditory, visual and kinetic learners can access it easily. This means giving information in verbal form and discussing it; using diagrams, pictures, video clips and models, and offering, where possible, 'hands-on' experiences such as inviting parents to put a life-sized doll through a model pelvis to illustrate the twists and turns the baby makes and how gravity can assist his progress.

> In order for information to be retained, it must be relevant; it must relate to parents' own experiences or experiences they have heard about, and it needs to be presented in a variety of ways so that auditory, visual and kinetic learners can access it easily.

Parents attending early parenting sessions are not training to be midwives. It is a useful exercise for educators to ask themselves what are the most vital pieces of information they would want parents to have if they could say only three things to them to prepare them for having their baby.

Many parents will have read widely about labour and birth, and will almost certainly have been talking to friends who have babies about what giving birth is like. The educator needs to build on the information that the group already holds. By eliciting information, s/he can then identify where the gaps in parents' knowledge lie, and also whether they have got hold of incorrect or misleading information:

- What have you heard about [for example] how labour starts; when to go to the birth centre/hospital; epidurals; pushing the baby out; delivery of the placenta?
- Did you also know that...?
- Is there anything else you want to know?
- You might find the following leaflets/websites interesting.

A model for information sharing/giving

Firstly: ask the group what they already know about the topic
Secondly: add any *essential* information that appears to be lacking
Thirdly: ask if there is anything else parents want to know
Finally: signpost them to further information

Birth hormones and the environment

Education for labour and birth should include discussion of how the hormones of labour – oxytocin, adrenalin and prolactin – work with or against each other in the different stages of labour, to facilitate or impede its progress. Understanding how birth hormones work helps women and their partners comprehend how important the environment of labour is. The educator can initiate a discussion on the significance of women having a safe space in which to labour and give birth. Asking couples to consider the conditions under which a cat, for example, chooses to birth will yield ideas about the importance of privacy, warmth, darkness and a sense of security. Like cats, women are mammals and in order to be able to tune into their instinctive understanding of how to give birth, they need the same kind of conditions as cats do to ensure the correct balance of birthing hormones. Oxytocin flows best when women feel safe, when their privacy is guaranteed and when they are unobserved except by those whom they choose to have near them. Discussion of the impact of the environment may persuade some couples to stay at home longer, where the conditions necessary for straightforward labour are generally more conducive than in a birth institution.

The educator can also help parents think about items that they might take from home to hospital or the birth centre in order to personalise the institutional environment and thereby increase their confidence that the act of giving birth is a normal human activity rather than one requiring 'the medical gaze'. The mother may prefer, for example, to have her own pillows to lean on, brought from home. Fathers and partners can be encouraged to see that they have an important role in creating a 'nest' for the labouring woman, protecting her privacy and shielding her from intrusive questioning and routine checks by health professionals. They can ask for mats and beanbags to be placed in the birthing room and for the lighting to be turned down. They can create a play list prior to labour so that the woman can enjoy music with which she is familiar and which can act both as a distraction and to promote calm. By finding ways to help the woman feel private and comfortable, and claim the hospital birthing space as her own, in so far as this is possible, fathers and partners increase the likelihood that labour will progress smoothly and without complications.

Early labour

The early part of labour, which often takes place at home, can set the tone for how the rest of labour unfolds – with the woman and her chosen birth companions feeling calm and in control or stressed and panicky. Therefore, educators may want to focus on this period in particular, inviting parents to consider how they might best control anxiety and prevent exhaustion prior to going to their chosen place of birth.

The decision regarding when to go to hospital or the birth centre may be of great concern to parents and requires discussion of the relative merits of the comfort of the home environment versus the perceived security of the medical environment. Providing time for couples to share with each other their feelings about how soon or how late in labour they wish to leave home is important; not all couples will have given thought to this and not all couples will realise that they may have very different views from each other.

> As early labour often sets the tone for how the rest of labour unfolds, it is important that educators help parents consider how they can control anxiety and avoid exhaustion while they are still at home.

Practical skills work in preparation for labour

A survey by Nolan (2008) of antenatal education noted that many women wanted more time in sessions to be devoted to practising self-help skills for labour, such as breathing and other relaxation techniques, active birth positions and massage. Some educators are daunted at the prospect of leading practical skills work. This discomfort may be due to lack of ease with their own bodies, a perception that couples might be reluctant to participate, not being convinced that self-help skills make a difference in labour, or unsuitable venues where there is insufficient space for people to move around freely. Yet labour and birth are fundamentally physical activities during which women must reach deep down into their primitive selves to understand how to birth their babies. For early parenting education sessions to imply, through lack of practical skills work, that birth is a cerebral activity, is to short-change parents and leave them unprepared for the reality and the intensity of the experience of labour.

It is the educator's confidence in introducing practical skills work, her will-ingness to demonstrate using her own body and her evident belief in the value of practising self-help skills that will carry parents with her – even those who may be reluctant to leave their seats and 'have a go'. Adults are pragmatic learners, so it is important for educators to provide a strong rationale for why upright, forward and open positions will help the baby to pass more easily through the pelvis, how massage strokes boost the mother's endorphins, and why relaxation techniques are linked through reduction in adrenalin to more effective contractions.

Mothers and fathers need to understand that gravity is the woman's greatest resource in the act of giving birth; that upright positions will make labour easier, contractions more bearable, and shorten labour. In addition, the educator can draw attention to the fact that upright positions decrease the sense of vulner-ability a labouring woman is likely to feel if she is lying on a bed and thereby assuming the role of a patient rather than being what she is – a healthy female engaged in a normal everyday activity. Fathers and partners need to understand the importance of the physical and psychological benefits for the woman of being mobile, able to choose her own positions and use the space in the birthing room as she wishes. The educator's role is to energise mothers and fathers for labour, supporting them to take control and claim the freedom to manage labour in the way that works best for them. Therefore, non-recumbent positions for labour, massage strokes, breathing techniques and relaxation strategies such as visu-alisation and positive affirmations need to be practised at *every* session. It is repetition that builds women's confidence in their bodies, and birth partners' understanding of how they can provide support. Campbell and Nolan (2019) report how highly women value regular practice:

> *It was the teaching it every week ... The calm ... repeating ... definitely increased my confidence.* (Kirsten)

> *What was really helpful was ... she always encouraged us to try different kinds of positions ... to see which position is the most comfortable for me ... It was easier to try different things [in labour] because I had tried them already during the course.* (Adali) (p79)

Parents will be helped to overcome the diffidence they may feel about practising active labour techniques if everyone is invited to try out the same positions, or massage strokes, or rhythmic breathing *at the same time*, copying what the educator is demonstrating. Humorous comments may be a strategy that some parents employ to cope with feelings of awkwardness and these often help the whole group and should be 'allowed' and enjoyed. Parents feel supported when the educator gives positive feedback about what they are doing and makes frequent links between the skills they are practising and how and when they might be employed in labour.

Practising non-recumbent positions for labour, massage strokes, breathing techniques and relaxation strategies at *every* session builds women's confidence in their bodies, and birth partners' understanding of how they can provide support.

Repeated practice of active birth positions is one of the most effective means of helping women (and their birth partners) enhance their self-efficacy, so that instead of feeling overwhelmed by the 'threat' of labour, they feel they have skills to cope.

Including fathers/partners

It will be evident from what has already been said in this chapter that fathers and partners are central to early parenting education in preparation for labour and birth. Women who have the support of a partner during labour have been shown to require less pharmacological pain relief and to feel more positive about their birth experience afterwards (Chan & Paterson-Brown, 2002). It is therefore essential for educators to keep the women's chosen birth companions at the centre of sessions. Good preparation can reduce birth companions' fear of seeing the mothers in pain (Wockel et al., 2007), and teaching massage and relaxation techniques to fathers and partners so that they can play an active part during labour is an effective way of increasing couple satisfaction after the birth and decreasing postnatal depressive symptoms (Latifses et al., 2005). In the course of facilitating practical skills work, educators can ask fathers/partners whether they will feel comfortable to provide support in the couple's chosen birth environment and what modifications to the environment might help them feel more relaxed. In addition, educators can explore fathers'/partners' feelings about various labour scenarios:

- How will you feel when you arrive at the hospital?
- How will you feel if the woman asks for a type of pain relief that she had previously said she didn't want?
- How will you react if a caesarean is necessary?

Fathers and partners should be asked to share their own or friends' experiences of being present at birth, with a view to helping them anticipate the anxiety that they might feel during labour, recognise the kinds of behaviour that characterise labouring women and have realistic expectations about the length of labour. Deave and Johnson (2008) found that men were not prepared for the personal distress that they experienced during labour. Nolan (2011) records a father explaining his experience of labour to his partner:

> *I didn't think it would be like this. I didn't think it would be so long. I didn't think you'd be making so much noise and I didn't know it would be so difficult.*

> (p97)

This labour was, in fact, a very normal ten hours in length, with no complications. In the UK The Fatherhood Institute (2014) states that teaching fathers techniques to manage their stress during labour and delivery should be a key element of antenatal preparation. Fathers and partners need to understand that the calm breathing techniques and muscular relaxation strategies they are practising in the parent education programme are as relevant for them, and will prove as beneficial, during labour (as well as after the birth), as for the mothers.

Educators need to keep the women's chosen birth companions at the centre of sessions. Good preparation can reduce fathers' and partners' fear of seeing the mother in pain. Enabling them to play an active part during labour increases couple satisfaction after the birth.

Positive birth stories

It can be difficult for educators to maintain a feeling of optimism about labour in any group of parents, whether awaiting their first experience of labour, or their second or third. Fear of pain, of 'loss of dignity' and of damage to or even the death of the baby, is partly generated by the long history of human birth and its very real dangers. However, it has also been fuelled more recently in minority countries by unhelpful media attention and by the removal of birth since the 1970s from the home to a medical environment with all its associations of pain, suffering and loss of control.

Sharing positive birth stories is an absolutely essential part of early parenting education. Such stories are rarely shared by mothers or fathers, for fear of being perceived as gloating (when all their friends and associates appear to have had a distressing experience of labour). In the context of early parenting education, positive birth stories gain a legitimacy that endows them with the power that they should indeed exert. A variety of positive experiences can be shared, including accounts of labour that required intervention but where the woman remained in control, and snippets of women's birth stories can be introduced by the educator to build a realistic – and perhaps unexpected – picture of labour:

> 'I was expecting agony or a show or waters breaking or something tangible but it was never anything like that with any of my [early] labours.'
>
> 'It was really long and really bloody boring.'
>
> 'Led to believe that early labour could last for days, but for me it wasn't even hours.'
>
> 'It wasn't as bad as I thought. Take your time to enjoy it; it's so beautiful.'
>
> 'It was terrifying, but also the most life-affirming experience.'
>
> (Anecdotes shared with the author by women she had taught)

'The surges are not stronger than me. They are me': a positive birth experience

I feel lucky to have had a positive experience of birth. Many stories you hear whilst pregnant are negative. A positive birth seems rare. This is not helped by programmes such as *One Born Every Minute*, which just show horror stories. I did pregnancy yoga from 22 weeks, continued running until 27 weeks and went to the gym up until the birth. My husband, Ed, and I did antenatal classes and online hypnobirthing modules. 'Hypnobirthing' is a bad name as it makes it sound airy-fairy but it is more about fully understanding what your body is going to go through and how to keep yourself in a positive frame of mind so that your body does what it needs to do. We learnt so much information from the classes and the online course, which made us both understand the process and what should happen. It makes complete sense that if you worry and adrenalin starts flowing, the oxytocin isn't going to flow. Classes also gave us the ability to question the midwives and ask about our options. I wrote a birth plan and 90% of it went to plan.

I woke at about 4.30a.m., went for a wee. On returning to bed, I felt something a bit warm. I didn't see the point of waking Ed as I thought labour would take hours so just put a maternity pad on and lay on a towel in bed. An hour later, I was in the bathroom again and Ed had woken. I said, 'I'm sure my waters have gone'. He was shocked and said it must have been the curry he cooked last night! We decided to watch the module on the early stages of labour from the hypnobirthing course again as a recap. I was getting a few aches but it wasn't too intense. By 7.30a.m., I was getting a little achier, so I decided to get in the bath. Ed brought me a cup of tea and a bagel with peanut butter. I was monitoring the surges [contractions] on my phone app and they seemed to increase quickly. After a while, my husband took over and monitored them as I thought I might drop the phone in the bath. I breathed through them with a quick breath in and a long breath out. Ed called the midwife at the hospital. She wanted to speak to me so I spoke to her on speaker and I think because I could talk, she didn't think I needed to go in.

We decided to go into hospital just after 9a.m. I was getting four contractions within ten minutes and they were over a minute long. The app on the phone was saying 'Go to hospital'. On arrival at the birth centre, they didn't think I was in active labour as I was too calm. I had a surge in the corridor and I just stopped and breathed through it. I wasn't making a noise. We went to a room to get checked and I was asked to wee in a pot so they could check my waters had broken. I said I knew they had. The midwife suggested she give me codeine [pain relief] but I wanted her to check me as I thought it was moving forward quickly. This was probably the most uncomfortable part of the labour. On checking, the midwife said I was 'paper thin'. I asked what that meant and she said I was 8 cm dilated and needed to go to a delivery room. I had the Red Room which was lovely as it is large and has some colour – a lot more homely. I was asked if I minded a trainee paramedic joining us; I didn't mind having her in the room as everyone has to learn. Getting into the bath straight away eased my backache. Ed talked me through the breathing and helped to keep me calm. Throughout the birth I thought of a positive affirmation: 'The surges are not stronger than me. They are me'. I used down breathing (short breath in and long breath out, pushing the breath down through my body) between surges to slowly push my baby downwards. When the natural surges came, I let my body do the pushing and when I felt I could, I helped to push down further. Through the birth I had a couple of sweets and dextrose tablets to keep me going. I thought I would use gas and air but it would have got in the way of the breathing and so I just used the downwards breathing. I changed positions from on my knees facing Ed to sitting on my bottom with my legs stretched out. Sometimes, the midwife had to get me to turn over so she could check the baby's heart rate but other than that, she left me to it. She seemed shocked at how calm and quiet I was. There were a few surges, which were quite stingy but I guess this was just because the baby's head was nearly out. Once the head came out, the next surge got the shoulders and he swam away, until the midwife turned him and he swam towards us. I picked Alfie up on to my chest at 1.51p.m.

I'm really glad I didn't have pain relief and that I could feel what my body was doing and work with it. It was a very positive experience. The only issue was that my placenta wouldn't deliver so I ended up in theatre to have it removed. It was strange being wheeled away from Ed and Alfie but I knew it needed to come out. It was lovely once I was reunited with them both again, even if I was shaking from the drugs in my body. I think it was a combination of my fitness, yoga and listening to my body that made it, overall, a very positive and enjoyable experience. I would also say that running the London Marathon in April 2018 was harder than childbirth!

(With thanks to the mother who shared her story)

Informed choice: interventions

Seeking informed consent to an intervention at the height of labour, be it an internal examination, acceleration of labour, administration of pethidine, insertion of an epidural or use of ventouse or forceps, is at best an attempt under difficult circumstances to keep the woman at the centre of her care, and at worst, a cursory glance in the direction of the legal requirement to seek permission for invasive procedures. While 'decisions' taken by parents during pregnancy may be reconsidered and overturned during labour itself, the opportunity to obtain accurate information, to discuss it with partner and peers and to reflect while not in pain or observing a loved one in pain, supports the rights and autonomy of the individual within the healthcare context. Transition to parenthood education provides such an opportunity. Educators may be nervous of spending time covering interventions for fear that doing so risks normalising them and implies that making choices about interventions will be part and parcel of the experience of labour. Parents, however, are often keen to learn more about medical procedures. Some will feel better prepared by having discussed them prenatally, although others will be made more anxious and feel less confident about their capacity to manage labour using their own resources.

As stated at the beginning of this chapter, the decision as to whether to include interventions in an early parenting programme deserves attention and educators should be able to justify for themselves and others why they have decided to include them or not. If the decision is taken not to include them, educators must be able to signpost parents to reliable sources of information, whether on the web, in books or via leaflets.

Parents-to-be, brought up on a diet of medical dramas and documentaries, often have a fascination with 'what can go wrong' and with the resources available to medics to manage or prevent adverse situations. It is all too easy to start a discussion about, for example, pharmacological pain relief in labour, and find that the discussion is ongoing an hour later, while time for practising skills for normal labour has reduced. Striking a balance, therefore, between respecting parents' need to know about medical interventions and the other important topics that crowd the early parenting agenda is a critical skill of the educator. Many parents will have read about pain relief in labour and there is no point in giving information that they already possess. Therefore, an activity such as a paperchase, where the group is divided into smaller groups and each one given a sheet headed with a pain relief choice:

- Gas and air
- Pethidine
- Epidural
- TENS

is very useful for eliciting what parents already know and any misinformation that they may have acquired. Each small group can be invited to list three things they know about the pain relief choice they have been allocated. After a couple of minutes, they pass their sheet to the next group and add two more points to the sheet they are now in possession of. A third and a fourth rotation follow with one more point being added at the third rotation and any questions being added at the fourth.

Groups are then invited to read out the six facts that have been written down about each form of pain relief. In order to ensure that the experiential aspect of each method of pain relief is covered, as well as the medical facts, the educator can ask the group if anyone has ever used the form of pain relief under discussion, or knows of anyone who has. This allows parents the opportunity to share their own or other people's stories – the stories that are likely to be far more impactful on their decision making than the hard facts.

If parents' list of facts for a particular form of pain relief is complete and accurate, the educator need do no more than acknowledge how well informed the group is, and ask if anyone has any further questions. If not, the educator should move on to the next pain relief choice, thus ensuring that momentum is maintained with a view to allotting an adequate, but not disproportionate, amount of time to the topic of interventions. It is, of course, important to ensure that a rich account of interventions is presented. A parent may disclose that her best friend thought 'pethidine was horrible and made her feel sick and disconnected from her body'. If no one has a different story to share, the educator may say that, while this is certainly some women's experience of pethidine, others find that it enables them to rest in between contractions. The point to make here is that the reaction to medication is highly individual and women who have never had pethidine cannot be sure whether they will find it more or less helpful in labour. Part of the decision-making process for each woman will be to take into account both the *known* facts about pethidine (given by injection often accompanied with another drug to manage sickness; makes the mother sleepy; could affect the baby's breathing if given close to delivery; may make initiating breastfeeding more difficult) and the *unknown* facts about how she, as an individual, will respond to the drug. Similarly, epidurals may, in the majority of cases, be effective in removing the pain of contractions, but women need to consider whether having a catheter in their back and one in their bladder, plus a blood pressure monitor on their arm and belly monitors to trace their baby's heart beat and contractions, will make them feel more or less in control of their labour. The means by which pain is relieved may be acceptable to some women and not to others. The reality of interventions is that every woman's physical and psychological response will be different. The facts tell only part of the story, and discussion in early parenting sessions needs to acknowledge the indeterminate nature of women's reactions to any intervention. It is not the educator's role to parent the parents.

> Parents do not want to feel patronised by the way information is presented or feel that it is 'sugar coated, as if they needed to be protected from the truth'
> (Newnham et al. 2017:55).

All educators, whether they are fierce proponents of straightforward vaginal birth, or strongly believe that medical interventions provide comfort and safety in labour, have a responsibility to examine their position, acknowledge it as theirs and not necessarily the parents', and reflect both in advance of the session and during it on the language they use. Midwife educators may also need to reflect on the alignment or misalignment between the remit of their profession to protect normal birth and the ethos and practice of the institution for which they work. In a fascinating article about 'mixed messages in childbirth education', Newnham and colleagues (2017:55) note how midwives in their study attempted 'to espouse the midwifery philosophy of normal birth, but this was moderated by a need to convey the fact that the institution [did] not tolerate any real trust in the birth process'. This therefore 'undermined the positive language that the midwives used to try and promote women's empowerment'.

Key points

Research and theory

- The majority of women would like to have a straightforward vaginal birth with no interventions

- Women who have the support of a partner or birth companion during labour have been shown to require less pharmacological pain relief and to feel more positive about their birth experience afterwards
- Women want plenty of time to be devoted to practising self-help skills for labour, such as breathing and relaxation techniques, active birth positions and massage

Into practice

- The educator's role is to help women and their chosen birth companions to maximise their capacity to work with the physiological process of labour in order to reap the benefits that normal labour provides for the baby and mother
- Early parenting education should enable mothers and their birth companions to reflect on the way in which they want their babies to come into the world
- Overloading and over-*burdening* parents with facts and figures is counter-productive as only a limited amount of information will be retained
- Understanding how birth hormones work helps women and their partners appreciate the importance of the environment of labour
- Educators can help parents to consider how they might best control anxiety and prevent exhaustion in early labour, prior to going to their chosen place of birth
- The educator's confidence in introducing practical work, her willingness to demonstrate using her own body and her belief in the value of self-help skills for labour will encourage parents to practise
- It is essential for educators to keep the women's chosen birth companions at the centre of sessions
- Teaching fathers, partners and birth companions techniques to manage their own stress levels during labour and delivery, as well as how to support the mother, should be a key element in antenatal preparation
- Sharing positive birth stories is a valuable activity in terms of making labour 'real' for parents

Note

In the Appendix are teaching activities, 'Perceptions of labour and birth', 'Labour and birth – dream versus media portrayal' and 'Breathing/practice contraction', which may be helpful in facilitating sessions focusing on preparing for normal birth.

References

Betrán, A.P., Temmerman, M., Kingdon, C., Mohiddin, A., Opiyo, N. et al. (2018) Optimising caesarean section use 3: Interventions to reduce unnecessary caesarean sections in healthy women and babies. *The Lancet*, 392:1358-1368.

Brownlee, S., Chalkidou, K., Doust, J., Elsshaug, A.G., Glasziou, P. et al. (2017) Evidence for overuse of medical services around the world. *The Lancet*, 390(10090):156-168.

Buckley, S.J. (2015) Executive summary of hormonal physiology of childbearing: Evidence and implications for women, babies and maternity care. *The Journal of Perinatal Education*, 24(3):145-153.

Campbell, V., Nolan, M.L. (2019) 'It definitely made a difference': A grounded theory study of yoga for pregnancy and women's self-efficacy for labour. *Midwifery*, 68:74-83.

Care Quality Commission (2015) *Survey of Women's Experiences of Maternity Care*. Care Quality Commission. Available at: www.cqc.org.uk/sites/default/files/20151215_mat15_statistical_release.pdf (accessed 23 November 2019).

Chan, K.L., Paterson-Brown, S. (2002) How do fathers feel after accompanying their partners in labour and delivery? *Journal of Obstetrics and Gynaecology*, 22(1):11-15.

Deave, T., Johnson, D. (2008) The transition to parenthood: what does it mean for fathers? *Journal of Advanced Nursing*, 63(6):626-633.

Dick-Read, G. (1942) *Childbirth Without Fear*. London: William Heinemann.

Jackson, P. (2014) Education for a calm birth. *International Journal of Birth and Parent Education*, 1(2):13-14.

Kassebaum, N.J., Bertozzi-Villa, A., Coggeshall, M.S., Shackelford, K.A., Steiner, C. et al. (2014) Global, regional, and national levels and causes of maternal mortality during 1990-2013: A systematic analysis for the Global Burden of Disease Study 2013. *The Lancet*, 384(9947):980-1004.

Latifses, V., Estroff, D.B., Field, T., Bush, J.P. (2005) Fathers massaging and relaxing their pregnant wives lowered anxiety and facilitated marital adjustment. *Journal of Bodywork and Movement Therapies*, 9(4):277-282.

NCT/RCM/RCOG (2007) *Making Normal Birth a Reality: Consensus Statement from the Maternity Care Working Party*. Available at: www.rcm.org.uk/sites/default/files/NormalBirthConsensusStatement.pdf (accessed 5 February 2019).

Newnham, E., McKellar, L., Pincombe, J. (2017) 'It's your body, but...' Mixed messages in childbirth education: Findings from a hospital ethnography. *Midwifery*, 55:53-59.

Nolan, M.L. (2008) Antenatal survey (1) What do women want? *The Practising Midwife*, 11(1):26-28.

Nolan, M.L. (2011) *Home Birth: The Politics of Difficult Choices*. London: Routledge.

O'Mahoney, F., Hofmeyr, G.J., Menon, V. (2010) Choice of instruments for assisted vaginal delivery. *Cochrane Systematic Review*. Available at: www.cochranelibrary.com/cdsr/doi/10.1002/14651858.CD005455.pub2/abstract (accessed 5 February 2019).

Sandall, J., Soltani, H., Gates, S., Shennan, A., Devane, D. (2016) Midwife-led continuity models versus other models of care for childbearing women. *Cochrane Database of Systematic Reviews*. Cochrane Pregnancy and Childbirth Group.

Smith, H., Peterson, N., Lagrew, D., Main, E. (2016) *Toolkit to Support Vaginal Birth and Reduce Primary Cesareans: A Quality Improvement Toolkit*. Stanford, CA: California Maternal Quality Care Collaborative.

The Fatherhood Institute (2014) *FI Research Summary: Fathers at the Birth*. Available at: www.fatherhoodinstitute.org/2014/fi-research-summary-fathers-at-the-birth/ (accessed 5 February 2019).

Uvnäs-Moberg, K. (1998) Oxytocin may mediate the benefits of positive social interactions and emotions. *Psychoneuroendocrinology*, 23(8):819-835.

Uvnäs-Moberg, K. (2013) *The Hormone of Closeness: The Role of Oxytocin in Relationships.* London: Pinter & Martin.

Wharton, K.R., Ecker, J.L., Wax, J.R. (2017) Approaches to limit intervention during labor and birth, Committee on Obstetric Practice. *Obstetrics and Gynecology*, 129(2):e20-e28.

Wockel, A., Schafer, E., Beggel, A., Abou-Dakin, M. (2007) Getting ready for birth: Impending fatherhood. *British Journal of Midwifery*, 15(6):344-348.

7 Education and support for home birth

Caregivers in the antenatal period have the opportunity to dispel myths and to offer birthing women an alternative discourse outside the cultural norm.

(Green 2016:11)

Research and theory

Evidence from the Birthplace in England Collaborative Group (2011) found that the safest place to give birth for women who are low-risk at the start of labour and who are expecting their second, third or fourth baby is at home. Even for women expecting their first baby, home remains a very safe place to birth. Yet this research appears to have had little impact on either maternity care professionals' or women's attitudes towards place of birth.

While birth has never been safer in the advanced economies of the world, this is not reflected in a concomitant confidence in women's ability to give birth without medical intervention. Indeed, there remains a strong conviction amongst women and many health professionals that birth is as safe as it is *because* it takes place in hospital and *because* it is frequently subjected to medical intervention. Even among birth activists, labour is seen as requiring at least the minimal intervention of 'support':

> *Vocabulary that emerged during the second half of the twentieth century has reinforced our cultural conditioning. Among groups promoting 'natural childbirth', certain terms became popular. A 'coach' is a guide bringing her (his) expertise. The need for 'emotional support' implies that to give birth, a woman needs some energy brought by somebody else. In the medical literature, the term 'labour management' is widely used. The terms 'coaching' and 'management' express the same way of thinking.*
>
> (Odent 2015:10-11)

The need for 'support' during a process that has been perceived by women for centuries as physically and emotionally challenging - because it is - has increasingly been interpreted as the need for *medical* support and this conviction is underpinned by a largely unquestioning regard for what Brigitte Jordan famously described as 'authoritative knowledge' (1997), the 'authority' being that of doctors and, to a lesser degree, of midwives. As the territory of doctors and midwives is the hospital, women have increasingly had to access the support they crave within a medical model of care.

National healthcare policies have, until very recently, strongly supported the choice of hospital as place of birth and reinforced the authority of the medical profession and the perception that birth is beyond the capacity of most women to manage on their own. The 1970 Peel Report published by the Department of Health and Social Services advised that every woman should give birth in hospital. Yet this was advice based on misinformation, as clearly demonstrated by Marjorie Tew in her ground-breaking book, *Safer Childbirth? A Critical History of Maternity Care* (1990). Tew notes wryly in her preface that:

> Far from being a record of conquering idealism, the realization of an advance in human welfare through the application of scientific knowledge to improve the natural process of birth by an altruistic profession with good reason to believe in the rightness of its methods, it turns out to be a record of the successful denial and concealment of extensive and unanimous evidence that obstetric intervention only rarely improves the natural process.
>
> (pvii)

By the time Tew published her book, the tide of medical intervention in childbirth had reached such a volume and strength that it was hard for most women and their families to imagine that birth in hospital might carry any dangers at all, or that childbirth could possibly be both safer and more satisfying in less technologically driven environments such as midwife-led units or their own homes.

The caesarean section rate in the UK has been climbing over the last thirty years from 12% in 1990 (Parliamentary Office of Science and Technology, 2002) to 28% in May 2017 (NHS Digital, 2017). It seems unlikely that a caesarean section rate of 28% in a largely healthy population of childbearing women accurately represents the incidence of pre-labour or in-labour complications. There are those who put the blame for women's choice of hospital birth on the media and programmes such as *One Born Every Minute* that frequently present birth as requiring 'heroic' action on the part of medical staff to save babies' lives. There are others who argue that the media does not shape culture but simply mirrors the culture that is prevalent and that rocketing intervention rates in labour and birth are part of a culture of trust in and dependence on medical 'solutions' to health 'problems' (Luce et al., 2017). Although the reasons for the increased use of caesarean continue to be the subject of debate, it seems likely that professional practice styles, in some countries driven by financial motivation, and/or by fear of malpractice litigation, are playing a major role even in the face of evidence that surgical birth carries risks for both mother and baby, and may adversely affect future pregnancies (Betrán et al., 2016).

> Professional practice styles, financial motivation and fear of litigation are driving high caesarean section rates in the face of evidence that surgical birth carries risk for mothers and babies.

During the nineties and through to the present, women and their partners attending antenatal sessions have expected to meet with at least surprise, and at the worst severe criticism, if they reveal that they are planning a home birth. Many of their peers will be mystified: 'What a brave thing to do!' 'What if something goes wrong?' are typical responses. Midwives may be supportive, but are often simultaneously nervous, and perhaps subconsciously hope for or look for reasons to persuade the woman that she should change her choice of place of birth and go into hospital.

At present, the home birth rate in England is around 2% (Office for National Statistics, 2016). Experts in cultural trends explain that it is not until a behaviour or attitude is manifest by 25% of the population that a tipping point is reached when the minority starts to influence the majority (Centola et al., 2018). It may be that this tipping point will be reached soon as new research into the hitherto not understood and not appreciated complexities of how the baby's adaptation to extra-uterine life is determined by what happens during labour and birth begins to influence midwives who are change agents and women who are leaders amongst their peers.

Into practice

A 2016 review in England concluded that around 10% of women would like to choose a home birth (National Maternity Review, 2016). They need encouragement to make this choice and to stick with it. The presence of a woman or a couple at an early parenting education programme who are having a home birth offers educators a wonderful opportunity to normalise their choice by being positive about home birth and ensuring that preparation for labour is always discussed in relation to the experience of labouring and giving birth at home, as well as in a midwife-led or obstetric unit. Every topic is considered in relation to the needs of the home-birthing couple as well as to the needs of couples who have made a different choice: topics such as how to use the environment to support the woman in labour, pain management strategies, the presence of family members, the moment of greeting the baby, and so on. Couples who attend an antenatal programme believing that home birth is 'dangerous' or 'not for people like us' and that it is disapproved of by health professionals may start to think otherwise and appreciate that home birth is not 'hippie' but a legitimate choice made in the interests of the mother, baby and new family and underpinned by the same con-siderations about safety as influence other couples' choice of a midwife-led unit or labour ward as place of birth.

Around 10% of women would like to choose a home birth.

Even if an early parenting programme is attended by no couples planning to have their baby at home, the educator can legitimately refer to home birth in the interests of fostering truly informed choice by increasing understanding (which may be limited) of the evidence around its safety. By sharing the facts and fig-ures with parents-to-be, the educator enables discussion both inside and out-side the parent education programme. Women and their partners will talk about what they have learned with members of their families, friends and other couples expecting a baby. When there is a vibrant, well-informed discussion going on at the community level, it is more likely that the 25% tipping point necessary for a cultural shift in relation to place of birth will be reached.

Honesty

Honesty is essential in tackling the subject of home birth. The educator must explain how the safety statistics differ for first-time mothers and those expecting their second or subsequent baby. The Birthplace in England Collaborative Group (2011) showed that, for every 1000 babies born to first-time mothers in hospital, *five* had problems. For every 1000 babies planned to be born at home, *nine* had problems. However, having a home birth for a first baby made it *less* likely that the mother would need extra help – forceps, ventouse or a caesarean section – to birth her baby. For mothers having their *second* baby, planned home birth also made it *less* likely that they would have an assisted or surgical birth, and was safer in terms of the overall wellbeing of mother and baby than giving birth in hospital. Sharing information about the likelihood of women needing to transfer from home to hospital during the course of labour is also important because couples are rightly concerned about this possibility:

> *For women having a first baby, there is a fairly high likelihood of transferring from home (45%) or from a midwifery unit (36–40%) to an obstetric unit (labour ward) during labour or immediately after the birth. For women having a second, third or fourth baby, planned home births and planned midwifery unit births offer benefits for the mother and appear to be as safe for the baby*

as birth in obstetric units (labour wards). The transfer rate to an obstetric unit (labour ward) from home or midwifery units is around 10%.

(Coxton 2014)

There's always a temptation for educators who are either very pro home birth, or very anti, to massage the figures according to their views on its safety and desirability. These views may have formed as a result of their own birth experiences, or their experiences of supporting women labouring at home and in hospital. Clearly, educators need to truly understand their own views and how they have been formed, and also to understand that they are just that – namely, *their* views – and not relevant to the decision making of the couples attending parent education sessions. The purpose of education for labour and birth is to present the evidence honestly without bias and then to provide an opportunity for women, and the person or people whom they are choosing to support them during labour, to weigh up what *for them* are the perceived risks of each place of birth. In hospital, these perceived risks may include loss of autonomy, not knowing the midwife who looks after them, being subjected to care routines that they may not want but feel powerless to refuse and being constrained by the limitations of the environment in terms of having an active labour. At home, the perceived risks may include not having medical assistance at hand if required and the distance to hospital should transfer be necessary (Lindgren et al., 2010).

> There is always a temptation for educators who are either very pro or very anti home birth to cherry-pick the evidence, or present it in such a way as to support their views.

Dispelling the myths

In a helpful article (Noble, 2016) by an experienced home birth midwife, a series of 'myths' that parents often refer to during early parenting sessions is presented with appropriate responses. The myths provide an excellent focus for discussion.

> 1.   Myth: Home birth is not safe.
>   Not true.
>   In fact, for some pregnant women, home birth is a safer option. If you have just seen a midwife in your pregnancy and are fit and well, you can consider home birth as an option. If you are a second-time mum with a healthy pregnancy, the benefits associated with home birth are that there is a higher chance of your having a normal birth; you are

less likely to have interventions such as episiotomy and forceps and less likely to need drugs for pain relief. Home birth is as safe for babies of second-time mums as hospital.

2.   Myth: Home birth is only for second-time mums.
     Not true.
     Home birth is an option for first-time mums as long as they have healthy pregnancies. The outcomes for first-time mums are better at home than in hospital as they are less likely to need a caesarean, forceps or an episiotomy, an epidural for pain relief or to have their labour speeded up with a hormone drip. First-time mums are also more likely to use water for pain relief, less likely to use drugs for pain relief, and more likely to breastfeed their babies for longer.

     However, the risk of an adverse outcome for the babies of first-time mothers is slightly higher at home than hospital. According to recent research, 991 out of 1000 babies born at home to first-time mums will be well compared with 995 out of 1000 babies born in hospital.

3.   Myth: Home birth is messy!
     Not true.
     There is surprisingly little mess! Every birth involves some bodily fluids, such as blood and amniotic fluid (water), but the majority of home-birthing families are pleasantly surprised at just how little mess there is and how quickly it is cleared away by the midwives. All clinical waste is taken back to the hospital. Your midwife will talk to you while you are pregnant about how to protect your furnishings and floors. We advise families to buy a dust sheet as additional protection for the sofa or bed. If you choose to give birth in a birthing pool, the mess will be contained and is easy to dispose of.

4.   Myth: Home birth is for hippies!
     Not true.
     Home birth is for everyone! Especially women who have had a straightforward birth before. Home birth is the preferred choice of many women and their partners, no matter where they live, what they do or their ethnic background.

5.   Myth: Hospitals are cleaner than my home.
     Not true.
     Giving birth at home reduces the risk of infection for both mother and baby. You are regularly exposed to the germs in your home – they are 'friendly' germs, whereas the germs present in hospital can be unknown to your immune system and therefore present a much bigger threat.

6.   Myth: I cannot have a home birth because my house is not suitable.
     Not true.
     If your home is where you are intending to bring your baby up, it is suitable.

7.   Myth: If I choose a home birth, I can't have any pain relief.
     Not true.
     Pain relief options are available; for example, you might wish to consider a birthing pool. You can also use gas and air, which the midwife will bring, and self-administered aromatherapy oils. You can learn hypnotherapy techniques for labour which your midwife will support you to use. You cannot have an epidural at home, because it is a medical procedure that requires an anaesthetist. However, research shows that women who birth at home need less pain relief than women who birth in hospital. This is thought to be because they are more relaxed, able to move around freely and have as many or as few people around them as they choose.

8.   Myth: What if it all goes wrong? Doctors and not midwives are qualified to deal with emergencies.
     Not true.
     Midwives are highly trained and skilled to deal with emergencies at home. Safety data support this.
     Every step possible is taken to reduce the chance of an emergency occurring at home. Only women with healthy pregnancies are actively encouraged to birth at home. The need to transfer to hospital is relatively common, but most transfers are for non-emergency reasons, such as a longer than expected labour or waters breaking and not being clear. In an emergency, midwives have first-line drugs and skills to cope at home until transfer to hospital.

9.   Myth: Even if I start my labour at home, the chances are I will end up in hospital.
     Unlikely.
     What is important is that you are in the right place at the right time. There is always a chance of transferring into hospital should complications arise. Transfer would be either in your own car or an ambulance depending on the reason.

     - Approximately forty-five in every 100 women expecting their first baby transfer.
     - Approximately twelve in every 100 women expecting their second or subsequent baby transfer.

     Very few transfers are for blue-light emergencies.

10. Myth: It is not good to birth at home with children present.
     Not true.
     This is a personal decision for you and your family to make. Children who are present at a home birth generally find it is a very positive experience for them. The midwife will recommend that there is an adult on hand to look after a child should s/he become upset. Whatever you decide, it's important that you feel free to focus on your labour rather than worrying about a child.

     (Adapted from Noble 2016.)

Involving fathers/partners

Considering every aspect of home birth from the father's/partner's point of view is essential. Fathers and partners can be invited to share what they feel are the positive aspects of home birth from their point of view, for example being able to choose the level of involvement they have in the labour, and what aspects of home birth make them feel anxious. Some fathers and partners will want to be with the labouring woman throughout her labour, but others may want to leave the room and have a break – something that is far easier to do at home than in a birth centre or in hospital. Couples can be given the opportunity to talk to each other about their feelings and what they want and expect from each other.

Birth stories

Birth stories support discussion about home birth, and can be used to reveal the many different circumstances of families who choose home birth, and to illustrate how birth plans may or may not work out as anticipated.

Home birth: mental preparation is important

I always remember that first midwife appointment where they fill out your green maternity notes with you. On the front there was a box for 'planned place of birth'. I knew I wanted to try to labour at home and when I told my midwife I'd like to try this, she seemed momentarily surprised but nevertheless wholeheartedly supportive.

I was so lucky that every single person I met throughout my pregnancy had an equally positive attitude to home birth, and that gave me so much confidence that it was something I could actually do. I really loved the idea of being able to go in my own shower afterwards and be in an environment that was familiar to me and my husband.

As a person with quite a busy mind, the preparation involved really helped me to feel in control. I was mindful that the most important job a midwife has is ensuring the safety of those in her care and I'd prepared myself for the possibility that I might end up in an ambulance if at any point things got a bit tricky. This included having a 'birth-day bag' packed with everything we needed ready for wherever we ended up.

A few weeks before I was due, my midwife turned up with a box containing everything we needed for birth and a couple of cans of gas and air. I bought some cheap shower curtains from the supermarket to protect the floors and some home comforts – a hot water bottle, some essential oils and sweets, isotonic drinks and nuts for energy. By this time, I was well and truly nesting and had already baked a big batch of cakes for the midwives and had cleaned the house from top to bottom. We were ready.

The day of Alice's birth was one of the most wonderful, surreal moments I've ever experienced. I remember getting into bed at about 11p.m. a couple of days before her due date and feeling a massive pop as my waters broke. Knowing I was going to meet my baby was so exciting and my husband and I laid out the sheets, put bunting on the fence out-side (to help the midwives find the house easily) and sorted everything we needed in the house.

At about 1a.m., I went for a shower and then set about keeping active, marching up and down the stairs and using a birthing ball. I spoke to the labour team on the phone and my on-call midwife was happy with how my contractions were progressing and how calm everything was.

At about 3a.m., things started to get a little more intense and I ran a bath. I remember turning over and over in the water as I breathed through the contractions. I still didn't really feel things were painful enough to be established labour but my husband persuaded me we really should call the midwife and get her to come over.

The midwife arrived at about 4a.m. and found me sitting on the loo, trying to hold back the urge to push. She coaxed me into the bedroom and on examining me discovered I was pretty much ready to deliver. I couldn't quite believe it but got ready on the floor to push baby out into the world. I don't remember feeling scared at all but just very calm and pretty excited about what my body was about to do.

The midwife hooked up the gas and air for me and gave me some instructions, including trying to hold baby in position between contractions as I crouched on all fours. I distinctly remember our second midwife turning up and offering to make her colleague a cup of tea between pushes.

I heard my baby cry before I saw her. As she let out her first wail, I gave one last push and the midwives passed her to me through my legs at just after 5a.m. I remember kneeling with the biggest smile on my face looking at this tiny red screaming child that I already felt so much love and protection for. Seeing my husband gently hold her for the first time was so touching and I was so happy that he had that time with her whilst I got cleaned up and dressed.

The midwives that night were amazing. They cleared everything away so quickly and we all sat round the kitchen table with a cuppa and some cake whilst I tried to take everything in.

It's absolutely true that the mental preparation you do for birth is as important as the physical act. In having supportive, continuous care throughout, and plenty of realistic advice, I felt really empowered in the choice that I'd made to have my baby at home.

(With thanks to the mother who shared her story)

In a birth education group run specifically for home birth mothers and couples, a story such as this provides plenty of material for discussion and stimulates questions that parents might not otherwise have thought to ask. The story injects realism into the session and contributes to effective emotional as well as practical preparation for the home birth journey.

Key points

Research and theory

- UK figures from 2016 suggest that around 10% of women would like to choose a home birth

Into practice

- Educators have a wonderful opportunity to normalise home birth by being positive about it and ensuring that preparation for labour is always discussed in relation to the experience of labouring and giving birth at home as well as in a midwife-led or obstetric unit
- Educators need to explore their own views on home birth and understand that they are not relevant to the decision making of the couples attending parenting education sessions
- The purpose of education for labour and birth is to present the evidence without bias and then to provide an opportunity for women, and the person or people whom they are choosing to support them during

labour, to weigh up for themselves the perceived risks of each place of birth

- Honesty is essential in tackling the subject of home birth – the educator must explain how safety statistics differ for first-time mothers and those expecting their second or subsequent baby. Giving information about the likelihood of women needing to transfer from home to hospital in labour is also important
- It is helpful to elicit and respond to 'myths' that parents often raise during early parenting education sessions, such as that medical pain relief is not available at home

Note

In the Appendix are teaching activities, 'Perceptions of labour and birth', 'Labour and birth – dream versus media portrayal' and 'Breathing/practice contraction', which may be helpful in facilitating sessions focusing on home birth.

References

Betrán, A.P., Ye, J., Moller, A-B., Zhang, J., Gülmezoglu, A.M. et al. (2016) The increasing trend in caesarean section rates: Global, regional and national estimates, 1990-2014. *PLOS One*. Available at: journals.plos.org/plosone/article?id=10.1371/journal.pone.0148343 (accessed 16 July 2018).
Birthplace in England Collaborative Group (2011) Perinatal and maternal outcomes by planned place of birth for healthy women with low risk pregnancies: The Birthplace in England national prospective cohort study. *British Medical Journal*, 343. Available at: doi.org/10.1136/bmj.d7400 (accessed 19 February 2018).
Centola, D., Becker, J., Brackbill, D., Baronchelli, A. (2018) Experimental evidence for tipping points in social convention. *Science*, 360(6393):1116-1119.
Coxton, C. (2014) *Birth Place Decisions*. London: Kings College. Available at: www.nhs.uk/Conditions/pregnancy-and-baby/Documents/Birth_place_decision_support_Generic_2_.pdf (accessed 18 February, 2018).
Department of Health and Social Services (1970) *The Peel Report*. London: HMSO.
Green, C. (2016) Preparing women for home birth. *International Journal of Birth and Parent Education*, 3(4):8-11.
Jordan, B. (1997) Authoritative knowledge and its construction. Ch. 1 in: Davis-Floyd, R., Sargent, C.F. (Eds.) *Childbirth and Authoritative Knowledge: Cross-cultural Perspectives*. Berkeley, CA: University of California Press.
Lindgren, H.E., Rådestad, I.J., Christensson, K., Wally-Bystrom, K., Hildingsson, I.M. et al. (2010) Perceptions of risk and risk management among 735 women who opted for a home birth. *Midwifery*, 26(2):163-172.
Luce, A., Hundley, V., van Teijlingen, E. (2017) *Midwifery, Childbirth and the Media*. Basingstoke, UK: Palgrave Macmillan.
National Maternity Review (2016) *Better Births – Improving Outcomes of Maternity Services in England*. Available at: www.england.nhs.uk/wp-content/uploads/2016/02/national-maternity-review-report.pdf (accessed 19 February 2018).
NHS Digital (2017) *Maternity Services Monthly Statistics, England – May 2017 – Experimental Statistics*. Available at: digital.nhs.uk/catalogue/PUB30099 (accessed 18 February 2018).

Noble, S. (2016) Home birth: FAQs and myth-busting. *International Journal of Birth and Parent Education*, 3(4):supplement.

Odent, M. (2015) *Do We Need Midwives?* London: Pinter & Martin.

Office for National Statistics (ONS) (2016) *Birth Characteristics in England and Wales: 2016.* London: ONS.

Parliamentary Office of Science and Technology (2002) *Caesarean Sections.* Available at: www.parliament.uk/documents/post/pn184.pdf (accessed 18 February 2018).

Tew, M. (1990) *Safer Childbirth? A Critical History of Maternity Care.* London: Chapman and Hall.

8   Education and support for women with fear of childbirth

[Pregnancy] is a time when the woman's self-esteem and self-belief ought to be flourishing, enabling her to enter motherhood from a position of strength. It is not a time when she should be alienated by her own fear from the experience of connecting with others including, most importantly, her baby.

(Davies 2014:8)

Research and theory

Abnormal fear of childbirth is given the clinical designation of tokophobia. Some women are so frightened of labour that they choose never to have children, or delay pregnancy until the biological clock is ticking towards the twelfth hour and their own strong desire to have a child, or their partner's, persuades them to try to overcome their fear and embark on a pregnancy.

While extreme examples of tokophobia are easy to spot, it is difficult to draw the line between women who are 'normally' anxious and those who have crossed a pathological line. A certain amount of anxiety about labour, birth and motherhood is to be expected and desirable. Adrenalin brings the body and mind to attention, preparing them to focus on the challenges ahead. Motivation to achieve desired goals is heightened along with creativity in devising strategies for coping.

Research has tried to put figures on the percentage of women who are pathologically fearful. Studies suggest that about a quarter of women express fears related to childbirth during pregnancy (Rouhe et al., 2011; Haines et al., 2012) and about 10% suffer from severe fear which manifests itself in nightmares, physical complaints such as asthma and irritable bowel syndrome, and inability to concentrate at work or to relax and enjoy everyday interactions at home and with friends (Saisto & Halmesmäki, 2003). These are women who may ask for an elective caesarean section (Stoll et al., 2015).

> Women who are abnormally frightened of birth may dissociate from their unborn baby who is the source of their fear.

As many studies have shown (e.g. Van den Bergh & Marcoen, 2004; Howerton & Bale, 2012; and see Chapter 5), sustained anxiety in pregnancy threatens the wellbeing of both mother and baby. The mother's resilience is reduced if her cortisol levels are constantly raised, with resulting damage to her immune system. The baby 'learns' that his wellbeing is under constant threat and he will therefore be born with a tendency to respond disproportionately to every uncomfortable experience such as hunger, thirst, cold, heat and noise.

Women who are abnormally frightened of birth may dissociate from their unborn baby who is the source of their fear. They may also withdraw from social situations (Nilsson & Lundgren, 2009) where banter about labour and the early days of parenthood is a normal part of conversation when there are expectant parents in the group. Isolation further threatens mental health (Figure 8.1).

Women with elevated fear of childbirth are over-represented within a particular demographic comprising younger women (Gao et al., 2015) with low educational attainment (Salomonsson et al., 2013) and a history of abuse (Heimstad et al., 2006). More generally, women who lack confidence in their ability to labour and give birth (Toohill et al., 2015), who rate their health as poor and lack social support (Laursen et al., 2008), who are dissatisfied with the support provided by their partner (Toohill et al., 2015) or who have had previous traumatic births (Elvander et al., 2013) may also suffer from elevated fear of birth.

Women can and should be helped to manage tokophobia. The consequences of not offering education and support are that women put pressure on birthing resources as they are more likely to request epidurals (Haines et al., 2012), to have longer labours (Adams et al., 2012) and finally to give birth by caesarean section (Ryding et al., 2015).

Into practice

Education to enable women to confront their fear of childbirth can be helpful when provided by skilled and compassionate educators who support them:

> *To self-observe and create a new, more flexible relationship with their original difficulty. With an improved understanding of the causes and effects of their problems, psycho-education can broaden clients' perceptions and interpretations of their problem.*
>
> (Toivanen et al. 2017:9)

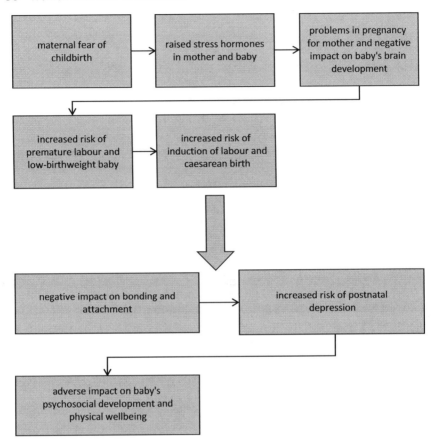

Figure 8.1 Impact of fear of childbirth on the mother, baby and their developing relationship.

Women with tokophobia and a history of poor mental health need specially focused support, ideally provided by health professionals who are not only experts in pregnancy, labour, birth and the puerperium, but are also trained in perinatal mental health. Women (and their partners) may benefit from individually tailored sessions, or sessions for the couple, which are repeated regularly throughout pregnancy.

For women who generally enjoy good mental health, and whose pregnancies are progressing normally, but who are unusually frightened of their forthcoming labours, group interventions provided by trained early parenting educators may be helpful. The content of sessions might include:

- Exploring the roots of childbirth-specific fears and anxieties
- Talking through previous traumatic pregnancies and births
- Devising and practising strategies for coping with fear and stress, including relaxation and mindfulness techniques

Naming fears

All women need to talk about their hopes and fears for labour and birth. For women with abnormal fear of childbirth, simply stating what their fears are, or trying to put them into words, may start the process of normalising and then managing them. Some women will enter into such a discussion eagerly; others may be silent because they feel that their fears are different from, or greater than, those of other women, or that they are related to specific aspects of childbirth which they are embarrassed to talk about, such as the possibility of soiling themselves during the pushing stage of labour. Educators need to draw everyone into the discussion, ensuring that high contributors do not dominate and low contributors are encouraged to share their feelings. Such a discussion makes great emotional demands on participants; it requires them to reflect on issues that may be painful or that they have never confronted before; therefore, the group needs to be small enough to provide a feeling of security and containment. Between four and eight women is probably best.

Inviting a woman who simply says, 'I'm terrified of labour', to identify which particular aspects of labour frighten her helps her to move from a situation where she feels overwhelmed by unnamed and unexplored terrors to a position where she can look at each element of her fearfulness and start to address it.

> For women with abnormal fear of childbirth, simply stating what their fears are, or trying to put them into words, may start the process of managing them.

Understanding the process of labour and birth

Toivanen et al. (2017) discuss the importance of helping women understand the nature of contractions. The educator can explain that pain in childbirth does not indicate injury as it does in other situations in life. Contractions 'advise' the mother on how to work with her body and use different positions to ease her pain and help her baby into the world. Movement is a core attribute of normal labour and is important in maximising the dimensions of the pelvis.

> *Women with FoC [fear of childbirth] may see childbirth as painful to no purpose ... their understanding of childbirth can be modified so that they see it as something natural, meaningful and manageable, thereby helping them to trust their capacity to handle and regulate the sensations and pain.*
>
> (Toivanen et al. 2017:9)

Response to fear and stress

Education for women with fear of childbirth needs to include discussion of how they respond to fear. Women will identify the common symptoms of stress – dry mouth, racing pulse, tension in various muscle groups, teeth grinding, headaches and abdominal pain. A progressive muscular relaxation activity, repeated regularly, can help women to recognise the difference between a contracted muscle and a relaxed one. Women can also be taught quick relaxation techniques (see box) for situations which require an in-the-moment response, such as giving a blood sample or attending hospital for an ultrasound scan. They can be encouraged to transfer these techniques into their everyday lives, monitoring their reactions to stress and managing tension through relaxation strategies.

Quick relaxation strategies

- Take a breath in through the nose followed by a long slow breath out through a softly open mouth (even better, make a low humming sound on the out-breath)
- Shrug the shoulders, and rotate them forwards and then backwards
- Ask another person to massage the shoulders briefly
- Stretch the arms upwards and then lower them gently down to the side
- Shake the hands out, then, holding on to something, shake the feet out
- Stroke each arm firmly from the shoulder down to the wrist using the opposite arm
- Scrunch up the muscles of the face and then release, ensuring the brow is wide and tall
- Smile

A discussion of group members' *psychological* response to challenging experiences in everyday life helps women explore their attitudes towards problems that they face. The educator can support them to explore whether they are the kind of person who tends to believe that 'things will turn out all right' or the kind who thinks that 'whatever can go wrong will go wrong'. Raising women's awareness of their usual mind-set is a first step to recalibrating their stress thermometers. The educator can introduce positive affirmations into early childbirth education sessions when relaxation skills are practised to counteract negative mind-sets:

- I respect myself and I accept myself
- I am doing my best and that's enough
- I treat myself kindly
- I am/am going to be a good mother

Affirmations for labour can be introduced in later sessions closer to the birth:

- I can do this and I will
- Each contraction is one nearer the birth of my baby
- I am a strong woman able to give birth
- My baby wants me to help her/him be born

Working with the body

Women with low self-efficacy for labour and birth and high levels of fear are stuck in a belief that they have no resources for managing labour. The educator aims to help each woman move from a position where she is adamant that she 'can't do this' to an increasingly confident position where she is willing 'to try to do this' and on to a commitment that she 'can and will do this'. In order to move from the first level of hopelessness to the final stage of believing in their own self-efficacy to give birth to their baby, the educator needs to show women '*how* they can do this' (Figure 8.2).

A key aspect of education for women with fear of childbirth is therefore practical skills work. Helping women acquire a variety of self-help skills that will ease the intensity of contractions and enhance their feeling of being in control is the essential accompaniment to providing anatomical and physiological information about how the body works to birth a baby. Skills work should be included in each session, enabling women to experiment with pillows, bean bags, birth balls and chairs in order to explore positions that will enable the pelvis to achieve its maximum dimensions. Relaxation sessions in which women can experience for themselves different techniques such as calm, slow breathing and counting breaths, visualisations and distraction techniques such as humming, chanting and reciting poems are essential to build confidence in women's capacity to employ them successfully in labour.

Relaxation and physical skills work is only likely to benefit women with fear of childbirth if they are practised regularly both in antenatal sessions and at home. Introducing skills in a single session, and never revisiting them in subsequent ones, is not likely to help women have an easier labour. Educators can encourage

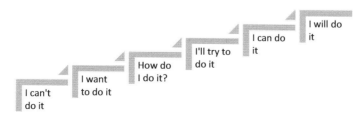

Figure 8.2 The self-efficacy staircase.

women to practise at home by referring them to online relaxation scripts, by providing diagrams of different comfort positions for labour to try out at home, and by texting them between sessions with reminders about the importance of regular practice, and offering warm encouragement to do so.

> Helping women with fear of childbirth to learn a variety of self-help skills that will ease the intensity of contractions and enhance their feeling of being in control is an essential part of their preparation for labour.

Confronting the fear

Based on the theory of cognitive behavioural therapy, Stoll et al. (2018) consider that prenatal education which incorporates 'exposure to the delivery room' may be helpful in addressing fears. The educator can arrange a visit to a delivery room where, with support and encouragement, the women can explore the environment, ask questions and practise how they might use the available space and furniture to make themselves comfortable during labour. It is obviously very helpful if the women's partners or birth companions can accompany them on this visit.

Further exposure to the feared event can be provided through watching a carefully selected video of birth. Seeing another woman successfully managing her labour, supported by her chosen birth companions and her midwife, may enable group members to identify the sources of their fear more precisely, formulate important questions, receive explanations about medical procedures and equipment and identify which aspects of the woman's behaviour helped her cope well and which actions of the midwife and of her birth companions were supportive. After viewing the video, women may feel able to start to put together a birth plan for their own labour.

Creative work

Davies (2014) discusses how creative work can help all women, and especially those who are unusually fearful of labour, prepare for childbirth. Painting, drawing and sculpting in clay may provide a means for women to express and explore their fears if they are not able to capture in words why they are fearful, or identify the source of their fears. Alternatively, women may find that expressing their fears in writing using a 'stream of consciousness' technique helps them identify what exactly it is they are fearful of, and why.

Artwork can be used to help women explore the kind of environment that would best support them to have a positive birth and what conditions would make them feel secure and confident to realise their aspirations for self-efficacy. Artwork also provides a means of anticipating how a positive birth would make them feel and how it would impact on their baby and their relationship with their baby. Facilitating such work requires a skilled educator who has had the opportunity to observe other educators engaging women in creative work and exploring with them the 'meaning' of their art.

Partners

Naturally, the woman's chosen birth companions need to be included in all or most of the antenatal sessions so that they are able to understand her fears and learn ways to support her to put into practice the physical and psychological skills she is learning in preparation for childbirth. The birth companions' support during labour is likely to be key in enabling the woman to persist with coping strategies, regulate her emotions and focus on her baby rather than on her fears. Loving attention from her partner during and in between contractions – kissing and cuddling, and speaking positively to her – boosts her oxytocin levels and reduces her fearful sense of isolation in facing the challenges of labour (Carter, 2011).

Previous traumatic labour

Extreme fear of childbirth may be the product of a previous traumatic labour. The woman's partner may also be traumatised if he or she was present at the time. Either or both may be unwilling to talk in a group for fear of upsetting other women and their partners. These couples may prefer to have a private ante-natal listening session with a midwife or childbirth educator, when they can go through the details of the first birth, and their recollections of what happened. It is often the case that fears are the product of gaps in the birth narrative and of misunderstanding what happened. The 'Self-assessment of maternal/paternal distress after a difficult birth' (see below) may be a useful framework for discussion during a listening visit.

Self-assessment of maternal/paternal distress after a difficult birth
(based on work by Penny Simkin and Phyllis Klaus 1995)

These are the positive things that I recall about my child's birth:

_____

_____

These are the negative things I recall about my child's birth:

_____

_____

During my labour and birth, I felt supported and cared for:

All or most of the time by _____

Some of the time by _____

A little bit by _____

Not at all by _____

These were times when I thought I was (she was) in danger of death or injury. During these times I felt (tick all boxes that apply):

worried ☐
frightened ☐
helpless ☐
out of control ☐
numb ☐
don't remember ☐
angry ☐
terrified ☐
disbelief ☐
near death ☐
detached ☐
other (explain) _____

These were times when the baby was or seemed to be in danger. During these times I felt (tick all boxes that apply):

worried ☐
frightened ☐
helpless ☐
out of control ☐
numb ☐
don't remember ☐
angry ☐
terrified ☐
disbelief ☐
near death ☐
detached ☐
other (explain) _____

I reacted to the danger to myself/my partner or my baby by (tick all boxes that apply):

panicking	☐
dissociating	☐
feeling detached	☐
cooperating	☐
resisting	☐
tensing up	☐
giving up	☐
don't remember	☐
crying	☐
trembling	☐
going blank	☐
falling apart	☐

other (explain) _____

Since about (how long after the birth?) _____ I have had the following symptoms (tick all boxes that apply):

sleep problems	☐
startling easily	☐
feeling alone	☐
panic attacks	☐
nightmares	☐
poor concentration	☐
flashbacks	☐
preoccupation	☐
irritability	☐
poor appetite	☐
reliving the event	☐
avoiding reminders of the event	☐
distress if reminded of birth	☐
detachment from my baby/loved ones	☐
crying	☐

other (explain) _____

I avoid things that remind me of the birth. For example (tick all boxes that apply):

- I did not return (go with my partner) to the doctor or midwife for the postpartum check-up ☐
- If asked about the birth, I don't want to have to talk about it ☐

- I didn't attend parenting groups or the reunion of the antenatal group ☐
- I drive out of my way to avoid going near the hospital ☐
- Other avoidance behaviours (explain) _____

_____

I feel flat or detached emotionally from my baby, partner, family and friends:

- All of the time ☐
- Some of the time ☐
- Never ☐

I feel I was wronged or treated badly by the following people in the following ways_____

I want and need these things_____

The educator can go through the woman's birth notes with her alone or with the couple, to enable better understanding of what happened, and plan for a more positive birth experience at the end of the current pregnancy. Following such an interview, the couple may feel able to attend group sessions for parents especially fearful of childbirth and thereby benefit from the support and shared understanding of others in the same situation. Alternatively, the educator may suggest that one or both of them would benefit from access to a psychological therapy, especially if fears are related to a history of abuse and require longer-term and more intensive support to address.

The benefits of offering women with tokophobia and their partners the opportunity to confront and manage their fears before the arrival of another child are multiple and important. Embarking on the next labour feeling calm and empowered offers the couple the chance of starting family life with strong self-esteem and their key relationships intact – between the mother and her baby, between the partner and his/her baby and between the couple themselves – and therefore ready to enjoy parenting and positive mental health.

Key points

Research and theory

- An estimated 10% of pregnant women are disabled by their fear of childbirth, suffering from nightmares, asthma, irritable bowel syndrome and inability to concentrate at work and relax at home

- Women who are abnormally frightened of birth may dissociate from their unborn baby and withdraw from social situations, thereby threatening both the baby's and their own mental health
- Women with elevated fear of childbirth are more likely to be young and have few qualifications and a history of abuse. More generally, women with tokophobia may rate their health as poor, lack social support, be dissatisfied with the support provided by their partner or have had previous traumatic births

Into practice

- For women with abnormal fear of childbirth, simply stating their fears may start the process of managing them
- Education for fear of childbirth needs to include discussion of women's physical and psychological responses to fear
- Helping women acquire a variety of self-help skills that will ease the intensity of contractions and enhance their feeling of being in control in labour is essential. Skills work should be included in every session
- Exposure to the delivery room may be helpful in addressing fears so that women can explore the birth environment, ask questions and practise how they might use the available space
- Painting, drawing and sculpting may provide a means for women to express and explore their fears
- Some women and some partners may benefit from referral for psychological therapies to help them manage their fear of childbirth

Note

In the Appendix are teaching activities, 'Perceptions of labour and birth', 'Labour and birth – dream versus media portrayal', 'Breathing/practice contraction' and 'Exploring mental health', which may be helpful in facilitating sessions for women with fear of childbirth.

References

Adams, S.S., Eberhard-Gran, M., Eskild, A. (2012) Fear of childbirth and duration of labour: A study of 2206 women with intended vaginal delivery. *British Journal of Obstetrics and Gynaecology*, 119:1238–1246.

Carter, S. (2011) The healing power of love: An oxytocin hypothesis. *Neuroscience Research*, 71:supplement e14.

Davies, L. (2014) The impact of fear of childbirth on the relationship between a mother and her baby. *International Journal of Birth and Parent Education*, 1(2):7–10.

Elvander C., Cnattingius, S., Kjerulff, K.H. (2013) Birth experience in women with low, intermediate or high levels of fear: Findings from the First Baby Study. *Birth*, 40:289–296.

Gao, L., Liu, X.J., Fu, B.L., Xie, W. (2015) Predictors of childbirth fear among pregnant Chinese women: A cross-sectional questionnaire survey. *Midwifery*, 31:865–870.

Haines, H., Rubertsson, C., Pallant, J., Hildingsson, I. (2012) The influence of women's fear, attitudes and beliefs of childbirth on mode and experience of birth. *BMC Pregnancy and Childbirth*, 12(1). Available at: bmcpregnancychildbirth.biomedcentral.com/track/pdf/10.1186/1471-2393-12-55?site=bmcpregnancychildbirth.biomedcentral.com (accessed 25 February 2018).

Heimstad, R., Dahloe, R., Laache, I., Skogvoll, E., Schei, B. (2006) Fear of childbirth and history of abuse: Implications for pregnancy and delivery. *Acta Obstetricia et Gynecologica Scandinavica*, 85:435–440.

Howerton, C.L., Bale, T.L. (2012) Prenatal programing: At the intersection of maternal stress and immune activation. *Hormones and Behavior*, 62(3):237–242.

Laursen, M., Hedegaard, M., Johansen, C. (2008) Fear of childbirth: Predictors and temporal changes among nulliparous women in the Danish National Birth Cohort. *British Journal of Obstetrics and Gynaecology*, 115:354–360.

Nilsson, C., Lundgren, I. (2009) Women's lived experience of fear of childbirth. *Midwifery*, 25(2):1–9.

Rouhe, H., Salmela-Aro, K., Gissler, M., Halmesmäki, E., Saisto, T. (2011) Mental health problems common in women with fear of childbirth. *British Journal of Obstetrics and Gynaecology*, 118(9):1104–1111.

Ryding, E.L., Lukasse, M., Van Parys, A. (2015) Fear of childbirth and risk of caesarean delivery: A cohort study in six European countries. *Birth*, 42:48–55.

Saisto, T., Halmesmäki, E. (2003) Fear of childbirth: A neglected dilemma. *Acta Obstetricia et Gynecologica Scandinavica*, 82(3):201–208.

Salomonsson, B., Gulberg, M.T., Alehagen, S., Wijma, K. (2013) Self-efficacy beliefs and fear of childbirth in nulliparous women. *Journal of Psychosomatic Obstetrics and Gynecology*, 34:116–121.

Simkin, P., Klaus, P. (1995) *Self Assessment of Maternal Distress After a Difficult Birth.* Available at www.angelfire.com/moon2/jkluchar1995/Docs/Self_Assmt_After_Difficult_Birth.pdf (accessed 6 February 2019).

Stoll, K., Edmonds, J.K., Hall, W.A. (2015) Fear of childbirth and preference for caesarean delivery among young American women before childbirth: A survey study. *Birth*, 42:270–276.

Stoll, K., Swift, E.M., Fairbrother, N., Nethery, E., Janssen, P. (2018) A systematic review of nonpharmacological prenatal interventions for pregnancy-specific anxiety and fear of childbirth. *Birth*, 45:7–18.

Toivanen, R., Saisto, T., Rouhe, H. (2017) Group intervention to treat fear of childbirth with psycho-education and relaxation exercises. *International Journal of Birth and Parent Education*, 4(3):8–13.

Toohill, J., Creedy, D.K., Gamble, J., Fenwick, J. (2015) A cross-sectional study to determine utility of childbirth fear screening in maternity practice – an Australian perspective. *Women and Birth*, 28:310–316.

Van den Bergh, B.R.H., Marcoen, A. (2004) High maternal antenatal anxiety is related to ADHD symptoms, externalizing problems, and anxiety in 8- and 9-year-olds. *Child Development*, 75(4):1085–1097.

9 Debriefing women following childbirth

Birth story workshops

A therapeutic group can provide a safe setting for emotional change.

(Toivanen et al. 2017:9)

Research and theory

In a seminal article published in the early 1990s, Penny Simkin (1991) describes the accuracy with which women remember the details of their labours and births, even many years after they have occurred. Women in their seventies could still give a minutely detailed account of how each of their children was born, and their recollections tallied with extraordinary accuracy with their medical records.

> *Women reported that their memories were vivid and deeply felt. Those with highest long-term satisfaction ratings thought that they accomplished something important, that they were in control, and that the birth experience contributed to their self-confidence and self-esteem. They had positive memories of their doctors' and nurses' words and actions. These positive associations were not reported among women with lower satisfaction ratings.*

(Simkin 1991:abstract)

Creedy et al. (2000) estimated that 33–45% of women consider their birth experience to have been traumatic owing to feeling out of control, experiencing intense fear, lack of support from their partner or chosen birth companions, loss of trust in midwifery and medical staff and an overall perception of not being listened to. A decade later, Alcorn et al. (2010) reported that as many as 43% of women experience childbirth as traumatic. Negative experiences during labour and birth impact on mothers' mental health in the following days, weeks, months and years (Ballard et al., 1995). Rijnders et al. (2008) noted that, three years after giving birth, more than one in five primiparas in the Netherlands looked back negatively on their birth experiences if these experiences had included having an assisted delivery or unplanned caesarean section, not having had choice of pain relief, dissatisfaction with the way in which they had managed pain, having experienced a poor relationship with their caregivers or fear for the baby's or their own life.

It has been estimated that 33–45% of women consider their birth experience to have been traumatic owing to feeling out of control, intense fear, lack of support, loss of trust in staff and an overall perception of not being listened to.

In recent years, studies have been undertaken to determine which aspects of the birth experience are experienced negatively by fathers/partners. In many ways, fathers'/partners' experiences echo those of mothers: that is, they may have been frightened that their partner and baby would die; they often felt unsupported by staff, lacked information about what was happening and felt helpless to do anything to assist their partners (Etheridge & Slade, 2017). Similarly, Inglis et al. (2016) found that fathers who considered themselves to be traumatised by their birth experiences had felt marginalised during the labour and excluded from communications between members of staff about their partner and their baby.

While there is a growing literature about posttraumatic stress disorder (PTSD) following childbirth, it may be that the term PTSD is over-used. It has been estimated that 3% of women develop PTSD following childbirth (Grekin & O'Hara, 2014) and, as yet, it is unknown how many men may be affected. What is certain is that many parents are deeply affected by their experiences, and may benefit from a 'childbirth review' (Sheen & Slade, 2015) or a birth stories workshop where they have the opportunity to talk individually or in a group about their feelings. A traumatic experience of birth is likely to overshadow the next pregnancy and labour. It may even lead a mother or a couple to choose not to have another baby, although prevalence rates for this are unknown (Baas et al., 2017). Providing women with the opportunity to understand what happened in their labour, to reflect with a skilled listener, or in a well-facilitated peer group, and to make plans for the conduct, both personal and professional, of their next labour, is a service that many women can benefit from. Such opportunities may also benefit fathers/partners although the research is not yet in place to confirm this.

Into practice

The aims of a childbirth review or birth stories workshop are:

- To foster positive mental health, and prevent depression, by supporting women to understand what happened during their labours, and to explore their emotions at the time, and subsequently

- To foster positive mental health through being part of a peer group where women can find companionship and support
- To enable women to choose to have another pregnancy, if they wish, with confidence
- To reduce fear of the next birth and to make it more likely that the next labour will be experienced positively.

Story telling

Women may self-refer to a birth stories workshop, or midwives may suggest to mothers in their care that they should attend if they are struggling with their labour and birth experiences. The offer to attend a session needs to be open to all women, whenever feels right for them to attend. Some women will decline the invitation because the birth is too recent, and the experience too raw, for them to talk about it. Some women will want the opportunity to tell their story and reflect many months or even years after the birth, or when they are contemplating or have embarked on another pregnancy.

It is helpful for both the women attending the birth stories workshop, and for the educator leading it, if the educator is accompanied by a colleague. If a woman becomes upset and needs to take time out, the colleague can go with her, leaving the educator to support the rest of the group and, as appropriate, to continue the workshop. Educators leading birth stories workshops need to be confident and experienced group leaders able to provide a safe and nurturing experience for women who are emotionally fragile; they also need to be able to recognise when women have serious psychological problems that require help beyond what the workshop can provide.

Before advertising birth stories workshops, a decision needs to be made about whether women will bring their babies with them or not. There are arguments on both sides. Babies are a huge distraction, both for their own mother and for other mothers. They may provide an excuse for group members not to engage fully with the (often difficult) content of the session. On the other hand, they may be helpful in promoting discussion of the perceived impact of the events of labour on the mothers' relationship with their babies. Some women will not be able to attend the session if babies are not 'allowed' because they have no one to leave the baby with, or because they are not prepared to leave their baby. The solution may be to provide a crèche, or for the colleague working with the educator to soothe and play with babies who require attention.

Following introductions and gaining the agreement of the group to essential ground rules relating to confidentiality, listening without interrupting and being free to leave the session for time-out if needed, the facilitator may open the discussion by exploring with the group their fundamental ideas about birth:

- How do you see birth in the 21st century?
- Do you consider it to be a normal, everyday event?
- Or is it a 'condition' and therefore requires the expertise of professionals, who can monitor it and intervene as required?
- What experiences during childhood or since do you think have influenced your current attitudes about birth?
- Have media portrayals of labour and birth affected you? How?

This is an introductory discussion that provides a platform from which women can move on to explore how their lived experiences of labour and birth did or did not meet their expectations. Telling the story of their labour and birth is at the heart of the workshop and needs careful handling by the educator who may invite group members to agree that each story should be told in five or ten minutes, depending on the size of the group. If the workshop is to last two hours, and there are eight women in the group, it is important to manage the time so that every woman has an opportunity to recount her story, and there is time left for analysis and exploration of the group's experiences.

After the stories are told, the educator can support the group to examine the impact of their experiences. How has labour affected the women's feelings about themselves? How has it affected their self-identity and self-esteem? Do they feel that what happened has in some way affected how other people see them, including their partners, family members, friends and the professionals who cared for them? Have their experiences affected their relationship with their babies? And their relationship with their partners? Are they the same people as they were before the labour or have they become someone different?

Schneider (2014:20) offers a list of questions for educators to use when reviewing childbirth experiences with women. She calls these 'meaning-making questions':

- What do you feel your birth experience reflects about you?
- What do you feel your birth experience reflects about you as a mother?
- What have you learned about yourself?
- What have you learned about your baby?
- What have you learned about the setting in which you gave birth?
- What thoughts and feelings do you have about giving birth in the future?
- What would you like to be different and what the same?
- If you had a friend who went through the experience you did, what would you say to her or suggest that she do? Can you do this yourself?
- Who in your life is able to listen to your birth experience, both the joyful parts and the distressing parts, and truly empathise and support you?

The educator validates every woman's feelings; however, she can also reflect ideas back to the woman to enable her to see herself 'from a distance' as it were:

*Are you saying that you used to believe that women are able to give birth natur-
ally, and the fact that your labour was complicated and required intervention
has disturbed that belief and your belief in yourself?*

*Your story seems to be all about your 'failure'. What parts of your labour do you
think you handled well?*

Recovery strategies

The educator cannot erase the events of labour which the women found
distressing, humiliating or terrifying, but having started them on a journey
towards greater understanding of what happened, and why they were so deeply
impacted, it is important to provide ongoing support and signpost towards community and professional resources. Every woman will be able to share something
she is doing to aid her recovery and can learn new strategies from the other
members of the group. The women may choose to continue to meet as a self-help
group without the educator. If they want to do this, the educator can make sure
that a date and venue have been agreed for the first meeting before the workshop finishes. Other self-help strategies that women may suggest are:

- Talking to the midwife who was with them during labour
- Talking to their partner about how they are feeling and finding out if he or
  she feels the same as they do
- Going out with the baby to meet other parents at baby groups
- Practising relaxation
- Contacting their GP if they feel that they need extra help such as counselling,
  cognitive behavioural therapy or antidepressant medication
- Getting in touch with the Birth Trauma Association (www.birth
  traumaassociation.org.uk)
- Or with PANDAS (Perinatal Anxiety and Depression Advice and Support)
  (www.pandasfoundation.org.uk/)
- If they are pregnant again, or planning another pregnancy, booking parent
  education sessions early and making a detailed plan for how they want to
  manage their labour.

If the educator is handing out a list of postnatal support groups, s/he needs
to check regularly that the information is up to date to avoid women feeling
abandoned and desperate if they are unable to get in contact with people and
organisations that they have been told can help them.

Every woman will be able to share something she is doing to aid her recovery
and can learn new strategies from the other members of the group.

Conclusion

The first labour and birth may be seen by mothers and midwives as providing a template for subsequent labours. Accepting this as true would mean condemning the many women whose first experience is far from positive to a childbearing future of distressing labours. Therefore, helping women, and their partners, work through and manage the emotions associated with a difficult labour is important for the family's mental health and for subsequent pregnancies and births. All women deserve a chance to talk about their labour with an empathetic listener in order to mitigate its impact on the relationship with their baby, their partner and on their next labour.

Key points

Research and theory

- It has been estimated that 33–45% of women consider their birth experience to have been traumatic owing to feeling out of control, intense fear, lack of support, loss of trust in staff and an overall perception of not being listened to
- Fathers who consider themselves to be traumatised by their birth experiences say that they were marginalised during labour and excluded from communications between members of staff about their partner and baby
- Having the opportunity to talk about their labour with an empathetic listener is particularly important for women who feel traumatised in order to mitigate its impact on their relationship with their baby, their partner and on their next labour

Into practice

- The aim of a childbirth review or birth stories workshop is to foster positive mental health and prevent depression, by supporting women to understand what happened during their labour and to explore their emotions at the time, and subsequently
- The educator leading a birth stories workshop should be accompanied by a colleague so that if a woman becomes upset, the colleague can comfort her, leaving the educator to continue the session with the rest of the group
- The educator needs to review the women's experiences by asking 'meaning-making questions'
- Women need ongoing support and the educator should know of community and professional resources to which s/he can direct them

---

Note

In the Appendix is a teaching activity, 'Labour and birth – dream versus media portrayal', which may be helpful in facilitating birth story workshops.

References

Alcorn, K.L., O'Donovan, A., Patrick, J.C., Creedy, D., Devilly, G.J. (2010) A prospective longitudinal study of the prevalence of post-traumatic stress disorder resulting from childbirth events. *Psychological Medicine*, 40(11):1849-1859.

Baas, M.A.M., Stramrood, C.A.I., Jijksman, L.M., de Jongh, A., van Pampus, M.G. (2017) The OptiMUM-study: EMDR therapy in pregnant women with posttraumatic stress disorder after previous childbirth and pregnant women with fear of childbirth: Design of a multicentre randomized controlled trial. *European Journal of Psychotraumatology*, 8(1):1-11.

Ballard, C.G., Stanley, A.K., Brockington, I.F. (1995) Post-traumatic stress disorder (PTSD) after childbirth. *British Journal of Psychiatry*, 166:525-528.

Creedy, D., Shochet, I.M., Horsfall, J. (2000) Childbirth and the development of acute trauma symptoms: Incidence and contributing factors. *Birth*, 27(2):104-111.

Etheridge, J., Slade, P. (2017) 'Nothing actually happened to me': The experiences of fathers who found childbirth traumatic. *BMC Pregnancy and Childbirth*, doi.org/10.1186/s12884-017-1259-y

Grekin, R., O'Hara, M. (2014) Prevalence and risk factors of postpartum posttraumatic stress disorder: A meta-analysis. *Clinical Psychology Review*, 34(4):389-401.

Inglis, C., Sharman, R., Reed, R. (2016) Paternal mental health following perceived traumatic childbirth. *Midwifery*, 41:125-131.

Rijnders, M., Baston, H., Schonbeck, Y., Van Der Pal, K., Prins, M. et al. (2008) Perinatal factors related to negative or positive recall of birth experience in women 3 years postpartum in the Netherlands. *Birth*, 35(2):107-116.

Schneider, D. (2014) Helping women cope with feelings of failure in childbirth. *International Journal of Birth and Parent Education*, 1(2):19-21.

Sheen, K., Slade, P. (2015) The efficacy of 'debriefing' after childbirth: Is there a case for targeted intervention? *Journal of Reproductive and Infant Psychology*, 33(3). doi.org/10.1080/02646838.2015.1009881

Simkin, P. (1991) Just another day in a woman's life? Women's long-term perceptions of their birth experiences. Part 1. *Birth*, 18(4):203-210.

Toivanen, R., Saisto, T., Rouhe, H. (2017) Group intervention to treat fear of childbirth with psycho-education and relaxation exercises. *International Journal of Birth and Parent Education*, 4(3):8-13.

10 Education and support for fathers

The loving care of a father is a foundation for his child's wellbeing and creates a life-long relationship.

(Global Fatherhood Charter 2019)

Research and theory

In the middle of the 20th century, fathers were, if Myles' *Textbook for Midwives* is an accurate guide to health professionals' attitudes, patronised and considered unequal to the demands of caring for babies. Myles tells mothers-to-be not to overburden fathers with tasks they may find distasteful, but rather to:

Allow your husband to share some of the pleasant little jobs for baby.

(Myles 1968:728)

Yet the world was changing. A letter from a father to *Mother & Baby* magazine in 1972 shows how fathers were fighting back against the stereotype so strongly evident in Myles' textbooks:

I strongly resent the imputation that we men are helpless layabeds who remain firmly rooted to the mattress while our wives dash about tending to screaming infants.

(*Mother & Baby* 1972:7)

The traditional view of fathers as breadwinners and disciplinarians was increasingly being challenged by men who wanted a greater role in the lives of their young children. Fathers' role was, in fact, about to change by necessity, as more and more mothers went back to work following the birth of their babies, and household and childcare responsibilities had to be shared. Gradually, fathers became increasingly involved in looking after their children (di Torella, 2014), although their contribution to the health of the mother in pregnancy, and their influence on the progress of labour, breastfeeding and postnatal mental health, remained largely unrecognised until research in the late 20th and the early 21st century began to explore these issues. A report by The Scottish Government, published in 2012, noted that fathers were asking to be recognised as part of the new family, from pregnancy onwards. The fathers surveyed wanted to have a voice and to be reassured that they were considered by health professionals as central to the life of their unborn and newborn baby (The Scottish Government, 2012:33). Far more is now known about the important part played by fathers in influencing the pregnant woman's and the baby's wellbeing.

Men are affected by their partner's pregnancy, not only emotionally, but also physically, undergoing detectable physiological changes (Bartlett, 2004). Levels of testosterone fall while levels of oestradiol (the primary female sex hormone) rise (Berg & Wynne-Edwards, 2001). Some men, in fact, experience similar symptoms to those of their partner, a syndrome known as 'couvade'. There are various theories that attempt to explain couvade, including that it is a psychiatric condition, that it represents male jealousy of women's reproductive capacity or that it is a response to actual biological changes in the man's body, as mentioned above. Symptoms of couvade appear to follow a pattern, starting in the first trimester of pregnancy, becoming less apparent during the second trimester and then reappearing in the third (Devi & Chanu, 2015).

> Men are affected by their partner's pregnancy, not only emotionally, but also physically, undergoing detectable physiological changes.

In the West, it is now usual for fathers to play a significant part in pregnancy, attending antenatal clinics with the mother and being with her during ultrasound scans (Redshaw & Henderson, 2013). Fathers are generally (but still not always) welcome at antenatal classes, although these are not always sympathetically scheduled to enable them to participate after working hours. The majority of women choose their partner, who is very likely to be the father of their child, as their support person during labour and birth (Fatherhood Institute, 2010). However, father involvement in the transition to parenthood is certainly not a global phenomenon. For example, in the Arab world, despite fathers' significant position within the family as the chief decision maker, including about their wives' healthcare, they do not trespass on the female preserves of pregnancy, antenatal care, birth and breastfeeding (Bawadi et al., 2016).

For fathers who are not physically present during the pregnancy, but are in spirit (those, for example, who are serving with the military or working for long periods of time away from home), the relationship with their baby is developing during pregnancy just as the mother's is. A Swedish study found that fathers' imaginings of their baby were as vivid as mothers', although men tended to visualise their baby *after* birth whereas the mothers visualised the baby in the womb (Seimyr et al., 2009).

The father's world changes fundamentally during pregnancy. His relationship with the mother is gradually redefined as the couple negotiate how they will maintain a satisfactory income and manage their home after the baby is born. The woman's mother and other members of her family may suddenly become far more frequently present in his life than before (Pollet et al., 2006). Yet while women are the focus of concern during pregnancy, the upheaval in the father's life may be far less well recognised, and he may have fewer people to whom he can turn to discuss his feelings (StGeorge & Fletcher, 2011).

Research lends support to the importance of including fathers from the start of the critical 1000 days. It has been noted (Hogg, 2014) that it is far easier to engage dads in pregnancy than to try to reach out to them after they have disengaged from their child's life. Fathers have, in general, a very low take-up of parenting support courses – the only training where they are more involved in parent education is in prenatal classes (Molinuevo, 2013). Early intervention during pregnancy may prevent the later development of problematic relationships in the new family.

> It is far easier to engage fathers in pregnancy than to reach out to them after they have perhaps disengaged from their child's life.

Fathers' key role across the transition to parenthood

Fathers have a key role to play during pregnancy in supporting the pregnant woman. Partner support is powerful in affecting the woman's adjustment to pregnancy (either for better or for worse) and more powerful than the influence of other people close to her (Pajulo et al., 2001). Consistent concern and interest on the part of the father predict the extent to which women attend their antenatal clinic appointments, and the degree to which they adjust their lifestyles to ensure their own and their unborn baby's wellbeing (Martin et al., 2007). Conversely, fathers' risky lifestyle behaviours make it less likely that their pregnant partners will choose safe behaviours. Pregnant women are more likely to report prenatal tobacco, alcohol and other substance use when their partner's consumption continues during the pregnancy (Mellingen et al., 2013). While some men who are perpetrators of domestic abuse may increase the level of violence against their partners during pregnancy, others are influenced by the pregnancy to change their abusive behaviour (Maxwell et al., 2012).

> Partner support is highly influential in affecting the woman's adjustment to pregnancy (either for better or for worse).

Postnatally, fathers have a significant role to play in breastfeeding (Everett et al., 2006; Tohotoa et al., 2009; Sherriff & Hall, 2011), with their support, or lack of it, being a primary influence on whether the woman has a successful and enjoyable experience of feeding her baby.

A review of interdisciplinary research into child welfare practice across the world (Zanoni et al., 2013) found that services were 'quite resistant to father-inclusive practice' and that their focus tended to be exclusively on mothers. A study of an Australian internet chat room for new fathers (StGeorge & Fletcher, 2011) found a persistent theme of fathers 'being left out' by services, which failed to advise them on how to help their partner, the baby and themselves negotiate the unknown territory of the first days of the baby's life. Yet it has been argued (Plantin et al., 2011) that if men are to be able to support their partner and their baby, they need to develop their identity as fathers and a positive role for themselves as soon as possible because 'paternal caregiving patterns that develop during infancy often persist and influence the way in which fathers interact with their children over time' (Hudson et al., 2003:228).

Including fathers from pregnancy onwards

The Fatherhood Institute (2010) argues that the antenatal period provides the ideal opportunity to engage with fathers. The transition to parenthood is a time when men are experiencing immense changes in their lives and are highly motivated to look for support (Rost & Johnsmeyer, 2014; Laws et al., 2019). They regularly attend clinics with their partners: 90% of fathers in England are present for ultrasound scans (Redshaw & Henderson, 2013); in Northern Ireland, 75% of fathers accompany the pregnant woman to at least one routine antenatal appointment while 90% are present at their babies' births (Alderdice et al., 2016). Educating fathers during pregnancy may yield substantial rewards for the family and society in later years as research has shown that fathers exercise a significant influence over their children's development, both while the children are very young and as adolescents. There is a correlation between fathers caring for their infants and playing with them and a reduction in behavioural problems in boys and emotional difficulties in girls (Ramchandani et al., 2013). The offspring of fathers who read and talked to them as babies and toddlers appear to have good concentration levels when they go to nursery, and to do better at maths (Baker, 2014). Verbal exchanges between fathers and their babies are predictive of pre-schoolers' social skills *independently* of the mothers' level of interaction with them (Feldman et al., 2013).

> Educating fathers during pregnancy may yield substantial rewards for the family and society in later years.

Family Included (an off-shoot of The Family Initiative, originating in Australia) has as its mission to make visible research that demonstrates convincingly that family-inclusive healthcare, and especially *father*-inclusive healthcare, improves women's access to health facilities, maternal mental health, infant nutrition and family planning:

> *This is because the family is the most influential agent over ... decisions and, if the family is well informed, decisions are better.*
>
> (Family Included: undated)

A recent report on the maternity services in England (Better Births, 2016:16) also repeatedly placed an emphasis on making maternity care family-inclusive:

> *For mothers and the wider family, pregnancy may be the first time they have sustained contact with health services and so presents the ideal opportunity to influence their life style and to maximize their life chances. It is therefore vital that families in England are supported by high quality maternity services which cater for their needs and support them to begin their new lives together.* (author's underlining)

Marginalisation of fathers presents three problems according to Clapton (2014:1):

1. It suggests that fathers are optional in children's lives, and don't contribute to children's wellbeing.
2. It is detrimental to mothers as it over-burdens them with sole rather than shared responsibility.
3. It dissuades take-up of and participation in services by fathers and pushes men to accept a diminished role in the life of their families.

More than forty years ago, Uri Bronfenbrenner (1974:35) lamented the lack of attention given to educating and supporting fathers to take their rightful place in family life:

> *It is a reflection of the narrow view our society holds of the nature and status of the paternal role, particularly in relation to young children, that the father has not been considered as an important target of intervention efforts, although his actual and potential effect on the development of the child may be as great or greater than the mother's.*

There is no doubt that the majority of fathers are as committed as mothers to raising children who will make a positive contribution in the world and who have

If educators provide information, advice and support to fathers

Fathers will understand more about the role they can play in caring for their baby

And about the impact of the transition to parenthood on their partner, themselves and their relationship

And therefore feel more confident as a father/partner, more valued and better prepared to meet the challenges of parenthood

As a result, they will be in a better position to provide sensitive care to their baby and emotional support to the mother. The baby will benefit from growing up in a nurturing environment where his or her mother feels supported

Figure 10.1 Logic model for education of fathers.

a sense of purpose and responsibility. It is therefore the responsibility of parent educators to support them in their fathering.

Into practice

As has already been noted, it is during pregnancy that educators have the best opportunity to reach out to fathers. The logic model in Figure 10.1 shows the beneficial sequence of events when this is put into practice.

Fathers want to know how to support their partners in pregnancy, labour and postnatally. They want *realistic* preparation for the challenges of early parenthood. Studies have found that men experience the first months of fatherhood as more uncomfortable than rewarding (Barclay & Lupton, 1999) and as disappointing, frustrating and overwhelming (McKellar et al., 2008; Premberg et al., 2008). Fathers want to know what to expect in the first few weeks of the baby's life and how they might feel, and to understand how their relationship with their partner might change (Deave et al., 2008). They want skills to help their partners and themselves (St George & Fletcher, 2011) and to be able to look after the baby (Matthey & Barnett, 1999). They want information about early childhood development and how to tell whether their baby is well or unwell (Buckelew et al., 2006). Overall, they want to be actively involved with their babies (Fletcher et al., 2008).

Studies such as The Scottish Government's *Bringing up Children* (2012) and *The Dad Project* (Hogg, 2014) have asked fathers how they would like information to be delivered to them. Fathers want concise information, relevant to their circumstances, offered on a need-to-know basis and in 'bitesize' chunks that are easy to understand and retain, such as:

> *Your baby can hear your voice even before she or he is born.*

They want *specific* information and *practical* tips on what they can do to be involved with their babies:

> *Take the time to talk to the bump; maybe play the baby some of your favourite music. This means that the baby will recognise your voice when he or she is born.*

Fathers-to-be like to hear the experiences of their peers and to receive advice from them. Therefore, sharing stories written by new fathers about their experiences, inviting them into early parenting sessions to chat and using videos that look at the early days of parenthood from the father's perspective are all useful strategies for stimulating discussion and making the point that the fathers are equally as important as the mothers. Educators can use extracts from books written by parents to provide a realistic appraisal of early parenting:

> *I remember walking into our little two-bedroom house and suddenly thinking how much we were going to need a bigger house to fit the clothes, the pram, the baby cot, the baby bath, all the other gear needed by a new family. As I closed the door behind me, it felt weird. It was as though the house had suddenly shrunk before my eyes.*
>
> (Williams 2018:47)

> *Barack and I studied little Malia, taking in the mystery of her rosebud lips, her dark fuzzy head and unfocused gaze, the herky-jerky way she moved her tiny limbs…We tracked her eating, her hours of sleep, her every gurgle. We analysed the contents of each soiled diaper as if it might tell us all her secrets…We debated whether Malia was too dependent on her pacifier and compared our respective methods for getting her to sleep. We were, as most new parents, obsessive and a little boring, and nothing made us happier.*
>
> (Obama 2018:191–192)

Early parenting education that aims to meet the gender-specific needs of both parents must include fathers as *equal* partners by using language that does not exclude them, teaching them babycare skills to enhance their confidence, ability and commitment to being a primary caregiver and providing them with opportunities to discuss their feelings about all aspects of new fatherhood.

Good preparation for labour involves sharing information with fathers, helping them understand what physical and emotional support their partners need, and listening to and acknowledging their fears. A well-prepared father has a positive effect on his partner's birth experience (Wockel et al., 2007). Teaching fathers massage and relaxation techniques so that they can support their partner during labour is an effective way to decrease postnatal depressive symptoms and increase marital satisfaction (Latifses et al., 2005).

> Teaching fathers babycare skills to enhance their confidence to be a primary caregiver, and providing them with opportunities to discuss their feelings about all aspects of new fatherhood, are key responsibilities of early parenting education.

Educators can encourage fathers to have skin-to-skin contact with their new baby, explaining how this builds the relationship between them. The use of video clips, of which there are many available on the internet (for example, on the Association for Infant Mental Health's site, https://aimh.org.uk/) can help fathers to read newborn babies' cues. Practical work with dolls can help them learn how to support the baby's head so that the baby can see her father's face clearly and enjoy a 'conversation' with him. Discussion in single-sex groups of what role new fathers want to play in their babies' lives is likely to elicit ideas around wanting to be included as an equal partner in the care of the baby and trusted to look after the baby on their own. Providing opportunities for couples to spend a few moments talking to each other about how the father wants to be involved with his baby may encourage women – who often act as 'gatekeepers', controlling access to the baby (Schoppe-Sullivan & Olsavsky, 2016) – to understand their partners' desire to play an active role in raising the baby. All of the ideas which are shared during sessions for interacting with the baby, such as singing, reading and playing, need to be set in a context of early parenting which presumes that both parents will be involved in these activities. Fathers' confidence will be boosted if the educator stresses that research does not support the long-held belief that there is any gender-based difference in terms of parents' ability to provide sensitive and responsive care to their babies (Feldman et al., 2010). S/he can also explain that a father's contribution to the development of the baby is different from that of the mother, and that he can offer the baby unique developmental opportunities:

When fathers sing to their infants, for example, they are likely to choose unconventional songs, or make up their own rather than sing traditional nursery songs...their exuberant singing being highly engaging.

(StGeorge & Fletcher 2014)

Fathers' style of play with their babies and toddlers tends to be more 'challenging' than mothers' (Collins et al., 2000), with teasing being a frequent characteristic. The educator can explain to fathers that their way of playing with and talking to their babies and infants has been shown to build children's confidence as well as enhancing the relationship between child and father. Video clips of fathers interacting with their babies normalise paternal involvement.

Babycare skills

A central part of any early parenting programme is to help fathers acquire practical babycare skills. While mothers need these skills too, of course, they tend to have far more opportunity to observe friends and relatives caring for their babies and to learn from them, and to have greater access to midwives and health visitors in the early weeks of parenthood. Prenatal sessions are the best opportunity for *fathers* to learn how to change nappies, bathe their baby, dress her appropriately, put her down to sleep safely and soothe her when distressed.

> *Group leaders should make it a priority to help men learn how to change nappies, bathe, soothe and settle babies. High levels of father/partner involvement with their babies are strongly linked with couples' satisfaction with their relationship and with family life.*
>
> (Craig & Sawriker 2006)

The educator can suggest that fathers might like to be the ones to practise babycare skills with the dolls, rather than the mothers, perhaps even splitting the fathers into a separate group so that they can 'have a go' without fear of criticism from their partners.

Breastfeeding

Given fathers' critical influence on breastfeeding, it is vital that they are invited to any session focusing on infant feeding and strongly encouraged to attend. One study (Brown & Davies, 2014) found that men are often excluded from antenatal breastfeeding education, although they are keen to receive information along with ideas about how to support their partner. Information can be presented in a manner that appeals to fathers. Information sheets that include concise, important and intriguing facts can stimulate far-ranging discussion about breastfeeding.

Breastfeeding fact sheet

1. Breast milk is mainly water – 87%
2. Breast milk changes flavour, depending on what mum has eaten. This exposes the baby to a wide range of flavours early on, leading to a child who is more willing to try new foods
3. It changes colour – it can be yellowish or blue/greenish depending on whether it comes at the beginning or end of a feed
4. It is different at the start and end of a feed – at the start of a feed, the milk is mostly lactose and at the end of the feed, it is mostly fat
5. A typical feed time is sixteen minutes – this is the average; breast feeds range from two minutes to one hour
6. Most women produce more milk in their right breast!
7. Breastfeeding has lots of health benefits – women who breastfeed have a reduced risk of osteoporosis, type 2 diabetes and breast and ovarian cancer
8. Breast milk is a 'medicine' – it contains antibodies that protect babies from serious diseases and anti-bacterial properties that help their immunity

It is vital that fathers as well as mothers know where to go for advice if breastfeeding challenges arise and where they can find support for themselves (Brown & Davies, 2014). Educators need to be able to signpost to websites and blogs specifically for fathers, and to local father support organisations.

Mental health

Information about and opportunities to discuss mental health across the transition to parenthood are highly relevant to fathers, of whom around 5–10% are affected by postnatal depression (Paulson & Bazemore, 2010). For fathers, as for mothers, the arrival of a baby is a time of adjustment with changes in their sleep pattern to accommodate, new roles and responsibilities to assume and new friendship networks to form. As with women, a previous history of depression renders new fathers particularly vulnerable to postnatal mental ill health. Owing to its negative impact on the family environment, paternal depression has been found to adversely influence infant temperament (Gutierrez-Galve et al., 2015).

Opportunities to discuss mental health across the transition to parenthood are highly relevant to fathers, of whom around 5-10% are affected by post-natal depression.

Educators can stimulate discussion about the possible difficulties of becoming a father and encourage disclosure of problems early on (Domoney et al., 2013). Sharing first-hand accounts can provide insight into fathers' experiences of depression and help tackle stigma:

> *Work was almost impossible now. I found myself starting to cry without even feeling it creeping up on me. It was the worst I could remember feeling ... my mental health was sliding ... I just wanted to do nothing, and that made me feel guilty. I started to avoid people, stopped going to training sessions as much as I should, and started to eat rubbish food. I was coming apart. I felt like I couldn't even express myself or make simple decisions. Just carrying on normal conversations was a struggle, never mind trying to close a sale. I wasn't just in a rut. I was about to lose my job, my company car, my wage.*
>
> (Williams 2018:88-89)

A recent review (Suto et al., 2017) of the potential of early parenting education to protect against paternal postnatal depression concluded:

> *Partner education during pregnancy may be able to prevent postnatal mental health problems, and support expectant fathers in their transition to parenthood.*
>
> (p115)

Even if the contribution made by early parenting sessions is small, it would seem reasonable that, in the absence of evidence that it is harmful, educators should continue to broach the topic of paternal postnatal depression and encourage fathers to seek help if they find themselves struggling in the postnatal period.

Key points

Research and theory

- The father's relationship with his baby is developing during pregnancy just as the mother's is. Fathers' imaginings of their baby are as vivid as mothers'
- The father's world changes fundamentally during pregnancy but the upheaval in his life may be far less well recognised, and he may have fewer people with whom he can discuss his feelings

- Father support is powerful in affecting the woman's adjustment to pregnancy and her lifestyle, and more powerful than the influence of other people close to her
- Fathers have a significant role to play in breastfeeding and their support, or lack of it, is a primary influence on whether the woman has a successful and enjoyable experience of feeding her baby
- Fathers often feel 'left out' by services and not helped to negotiate the unknown territory of the first days of their baby's life
- Marginalisation of fathers implies that fathers are optional in their children's lives and dissuades them from making use of family services
- Including fathers in early parenting education may yield substantial rewards for the family and society in later years as research has shown that fathers exercise a significant influence over their children's development

Into practice

- Good preparation for labour involves sharing information with fathers, helping them understand what physical and emotional support their partners need, teaching them massage and relaxation techniques and listening to and acknowledging their fears
- All ideas for interacting with the baby, such as singing, reading and mutual gaze, need to be set by the educator in an early parenting context which presumes that *both* parents will be involved in these activities. Video clips of fathers interacting with their babies normalise paternal involvement
- Educators should help fathers to acquire practical babycare skills
- Inviting new fathers to attend sessions is a useful strategy for engaging fathers-to-be in discussion
- Reading from first-hand accounts of fathers who have suffered from postnatal depression can provide insight into fathers' experiences of mental ill health and help tackle stigma
- Fathers as well as mothers need to know where to turn for support if breastfeeding crises arise
- Educators need to be able to signpost to internet resources for fathers and to local father support organisations

Note

In the Appendix are teaching activities, 'Preparing for the realities of early postnatal life', 'Finding time for each other', 'What do you want for your baby? What does your baby need?' and 'Exploring mental health', which may be helpful in facilitating sessions focusing on fathers' transition to parenthood.

References

Alderdice, F., Hamilton, K., McNeill, J., Lynn, F., Curran, R. et al. (2016) *Birth NI: A Survey of Women's Experience of Maternity Care in Northern Ireland*. Belfast: National Perinatal Epidemiology Unit (NPEU) with Nursing and Midwifery at Queen's University, Belfast.

Baker, C.E. (2014) African American fathers' contributions to children's preschool reading and math achievement: Evidence from two-parent families from the Early Childhood Longitudinal Study – Birth Cohort. *Early Education and Development*, 25(1):19–35.

Barclay, L., Lupton, D. (1999) The experiences of new fatherhood: A socio-cultural analysis. *Journal of Advanced Nursing*, 29(4):1013–1020.

Bartlett, E.E. (2004) The effects of fatherhood on the health of men: A review of the literature. *The Journal of Men's Health & Gender*, 1(2–3):159–169.

Bawadi, H.A., Qandil, A.M., Al-Hamdan, Z.M., Mahallawi, H.H. (2016) The role of fathers during pregnancy: A qualitative exploration of Arabic fathers' beliefs. *Midwifery*, 32:75–80.

Berg, S.J., Wynne-Edwards, K.E. (2001) Changes in testosterone, cortisol, and estradiol levels in men becoming fathers. *Mayo Clinic Proceedings*, 76(6):582–592.

Better Births. *Improving Outcomes of Maternity Services in England – A Five Year Forward View for Maternity Care* (2016) Available at: www.england.nhs.uk/wp-content/uploads/2016/02/national-maternity-review-report.pdf (accessed 16 February 2019).

Bronfenbrenner, U. (1974) *A Report on Longitudinal Evaluations of Preschool Programs, Volume II: Is Early Intervention Effective?* Washington, DC: US Department of Health, Educational Welfare and the National Institute of Education.

Brown, A., Davies, R. (2014) Fathers' experiences of supporting breastfeeding: challenges for breastfeeding promotion and education. *Maternal and Child Nutrition*, 10:510–526.

Buckelew, S.M., Pierrie, H., Chabra, A. (2006) What fathers need: A countywide assessment of the needs of fathers of young children. *Maternal and Child Health Journal*, 10(3):285–291.

Clapton, G. (2014) The birth certificate, 'father unknown' and adoption. *Adoption and Fostering*, 38(3):209–222.

Collins, W.A., Maccoby, E.E., Steinberg, L., Hetherington, E.M., Bornstein, M.H. (2000) Contemporary research on parenting: The case for nature and nurture. *American Psychologist*, 55(2):218–232.

Craig, L., Sawriker, P. (2006) *Work and Family Balance: Transitions to High School*. Unpublished draft final report. University of New South Wales: Social Policy Research Centre.

Deave, T., Johnson, J., Ingram, J. (2008) Transition to parenthood: The needs of parents in pregnancy and early parenthood. *BMC Pregnancy and Childbirth*, 8(30). Available at: https://bmcpregnancychildbirth.biomedcentral.com/articles/10.1186/1471-2393-8-30 (accessed 1 January 2018).

Devi, A.M., Chanu, M.P. (2015) Couvade syndrome. *International Journal of Nursing Education and Research*, 3(3):109–111.

Di Torella, E.C. (2014) Brave new fathers for a brave new world? Fathers as caregivers in an evolving European Union. *European Law Journal*, 20(1):88–106.

Domoney, J., Iles, J., Ramchandani, P. (2013) Paternal depression in the postnatal period: Reflections on current knowledge and practice. *International Journal of Birth and Parent Education*, 1(3):17–20.

Everett, K.D., Bullock, L., Gage, J.D. et al. (2006) Health risk behaviour of rural low-income fathers. *Public Health Nursing*, 23(4):297–306.

Family Included (undated) *Family Included: About*. Available at: https://familyincluded.com/about/ (accessed 17 February 2019).

Fatherhood Institute (2010) *Fathers and Family Health in the Perinatal Period: A Briefing on the Benefits of Paternal Engagement*. London: Fatherhood Institute.

Feldman, R., Gordon, I., Schneiderman, I., Welsman, O., Zagoory-Sharon, O. (2010) Natural variations in maternal and paternal care are associated with systematic changes in oxytocin following parent–infant contact. *Psychoneuroendocrinology*, 35(8):1133–1141.

Feldman, R., Gordon, I., Influs, M., Gutbir, T., Ebstein, R.P. (2013) Parental oxytocin and early caregiving jointly shape children's oxytocin response and social reciprocity. *Neuropsychopharmacology*, 38:1154–1162.

Fletcher, R., Vimpani, G., Russell, G., Keatinge, D. (2008) The evaluation of tailored and web-based information for new fathers. *Child:Care, Health and Development*, 34(4):439–446.

Global Fatherhood Charter (2019) Quoted in: *International Journal of Birth and Parent Education*, 7(1):34.

Gutierrez-Galve, L., Stein, A., Hanington, L., Heron, J., Ramchandani, P. (2015) Paternal depression in the postnatal period and child development: Mediators and moderators. *Pediatrics*, 135(2):e339–e347.

Hogg, S. (2014) *The Dad Project*. London:NSPCC.

Hudson, D.B., Campbell-Grossman, C., Fleck, M.O., Elek, S.M., Shipman, A. (2003) Effect of the New Fathers Network on first-time fathers' parenting self-efficacy and parenting satisfaction during the transition to parenthood. *Issues in Comprehensive Pediatric Nursing*, 26(4):217-229.

Latifses, V., Estroff, D.B., Field, T., Bush, J.P. (2005) Fathers massaging and relaxing their pregnant wives lowered anxiety and facilitated marital adjustment. *Journal of Bodywork and Movement Therapies*, 9(4):277-282.

Laws, R., Walsh, A.D., Hesketh, K.D., Downing, K.L., Kuswara, K. et al. (2019) Differences between mothers and fathers of young children in their use of the internet to support healthy family lifestyle behaviors: Cross-sectional study. *Journal of Medical Internet Research*, 21(1):e11454.

Martin, A., Ryan, R.M., Brooks-Gunn, J. (2007) The joint influence of mother and father parenting on child cognitive outcomes at age 5. *Early Childhood Research Quarterly*, 22(4):423-439.

Matthey, S., Barnett, B. (1999) Parent–infant classes in the early postpartum period: Need and participation by fathers and mothers. *Infant Mental Health Journal*, 20(3):278-290.

Maxwell, N., Scourfield, J., Holland, S., Featherstone, B., Lee, J. (2012) The benefits and challenges of training child protection social workers in father engagement. *Child Abuse Review*, 21(4):299-310.

McKellar, L., Pincombe, J., Henderson, A. (2008) Enhancing fathers' educational experiences during the early postnatal period. *The Journal of Perinatal Education*, 17(4):12-20.

Mellingen, S., Torsheim, T., Thuen, F. (2013) Changes in alcohol use and relationship satisfaction in Norwegian couples during pregnancy. *Substance Abuse Treatment, Prevention and Policy*, 8(5). Available at: https://substanceabusepolicy.biomedcentral.com/track/pdf/10.1186/1747-597X-8-5?site=substanceabusepolicy.biomedcentral.com (accessed 30 December 2017).

Molinuevo, D. (2013) *Parenting Support in Europe*. Dublin: European Foundation for the Improvement of Living and Working Conditions.

Mother & Baby (1972) *Our News*. February.

Myles, M. (1968) *A Textbook for Midwives, 6th Edition*. Edinburgh:E&S Livingstone.

Obama, M. (2018) *Becoming*. UK: Viking.

Pajulo, M., Savonlahti, E., Sourander, A., Helenius, H., Piha, J. (2001) Antenatal depression, substance dependency and social support. *Journal of Affective Disorders*, 65(1):9-17.

Paulson, J.F., Bazemore, S.D. (2010) Prenatal and postnatal depression in fathers and its association with maternal depression. *Journal of the American Medical Association*, 303(19):1961-1969.

Plantin, L., Olukoya, A.A., Ny, P. (2011) Positive health outcomes of fathers' involvement in pregnancy and childbirth paternal support: A scope study literature review. *Fathering*, 9(1):87-102.

Pollet, T.V., Nettle, D., Nelissen, M. (2006) Contact frequencies between grandparents and grandchildren in a modern society: Estimates of the impact of paternity uncertainty. *Journal of Cultural and Evolutionary Psychology*, 4 (3-4):203-213.

Premberg, A., Hellström, A.L., Berg, M. (2008) Experiences of the first year as father. *Scandinavian Journal of Caring Sciences*, 22(1):56-63.

Ramchandani, P.G., Domoney, J., Sethna, V. et al. (2013) Do early father-infant interactions predict the onset of externalising behaviours in young children? Findings from a longitudinal cohort study. *Journal of Child Psychology and Psychiatry and Allied Disciplines*, 54(1):56-64.

Redshaw, M., Henderson, J. (2013) Fathers' engagement in pregnancy and childbirth: Evidence from a national survey. *Pregnancy and Childbirth*, 13:70-85.

Rost, J., Johnsmeyer, B. (2014) *Think with Google: Think Insights with Google Series 2014. Diapers to Diplomas: What's on the Minds of New Parents?* Available at: www.thinkwithgoogle.com/consumer-insights/new-parents/ (accessed 13 August 2019).

Schoppe-Sullivan, S., Olsavsky, A. (2016) Promoting supportive coparenting relationships to engage fathers: Helping mothers to open the gate and stand back. *International Journal of Birth and Parent Education*, 4(1):15-19.

Sherriff, N., Hall, V. (2011) Engaging and supporting fathers to promote breastfeeding: A new role for health visitors? *Scandinavian Journal of Caring Sciences*, 25(3):467-475.

Seimyr, L., Sjögren, B., Welles-Nyström, B., Nissen, E. (2009) Antenatal maternal depressive mood and parental-fetal attachment at the end of pregnancy. *Archives of Women's Mental Health*, 12:269-279.

StGeorge, J.M., Fletcher, R.J. (2011) Fathers online: Learning about fatherhood through the internet. *The Journal of Perinatal Education*, 20(3):154.

StGeorge, J.M., Fletcher, R.J. (2014) 'Daddy's funny!' Fathers' playfulness with young children. *International Journal of Birth and Parent Education*, 2(1):11-12.

Suto, M., Takehara, K., Yamane, Y., Ota, E. (2017) Effects of prenatal childbirth education for partners of pregnant women on paternal postnatal mental health and couple relationship: A systematic review. *Journal of Affective Disorders*, 210:115-121.

The Scottish Government (2012) *Bringing Up Children: Your Views*. Edinburgh: The Scottish Government.

Tohotoa, J., Maycock, B., Hauck, Y.L. et al. (2009) Dads make a difference: An exploratory study of paternal support for breastfeeding in Perth, Western Australia. *International Breastfeeding Journal*, 4(15). Available at: https://internationalbreastfeedingjournal.biomedcentral.com/track/pdf/10.1186/1746-4358-4-15?site=internationalbreastfeedingjournal.biomedcentral.com (accessed 1 January 2018).

Williams, M. (2018) *Daddy Blues*. Newark, Notts.: Trigger.

Wockel, A., Schafer, E., Beggel, A., Abou-Dakin, M. (2007) Getting ready for birth: Impending fatherhood. *British Journal of Midwifery*, 15(6):344-348.

Zanoni, L., Warburton, W., Bussey K. et al. (2013) Fathers as 'core business' in child welfare practice and research: An interdisciplinary review. *Children and Youth Services Review*, 35(7):1055-1070.

11 Education and support for the couple relationship across the transition to parenthood

Although relationship declines are common for many new parents, they are not inevitable. Rather than taking a deficit view of this transition [to parenthood], it is useful to adopt a more strengths-based approach, identifying areas that help to protect couples from relationship problems.

(Houlston et al. 2013:21)

Research and theory

It is unwise to make sweeping generalisations about the impact of any particular event in a couple's life on the functioning of their relationship. Couples vary in terms of their pre-existing vulnerability to relationship breakdown, the degree of stress to which any particular life event exposes them and their capacity for adapting to new challenges. However, there is a considerable body of research to indicate that the transition to first-time parenthood is difficult for many couples (e.g. Lawrence et al., 2008; Doss et al., 2009) who experience the first weeks and months with their baby as a time of exceptional demands. Many struggle with exhaustion (Petch & Halford, 2008), role overload (Perry-Jenkins et al., 2007) and reduced time for each to participate in previously enjoyed leisure activities and for intimacy (Feeney et al., 2001). The birth of even a much-longed-for infant may therefore lead not to an increase in marital/relationship satisfaction, but to serious threats to its quality and its continuance. Couples in Western societies may find themselves largely unsupported. They may live far away from grandparents, or grandparents may be working full-time and not available to help with household chores and childcare, and friends and neighbours may not offer support in communities where 'community' is no longer a reality. Tiredness exacerbated by lack of support and a feeling of being overwhelmed by new responsibilities may lead to failures of communication (Huston & Holmes, 2004; Howard & Brooks-Gunn, 2009) and decreasing cooperation with each other.

Couple conflict has implications beyond the wellbeing of the couple themselves. For nearly ninety years, research has been demonstrating that conflict between parents impacts children's health and wellbeing (Towle, 1931; Emery, 1982; Harold & Congar, 1997; Houlston et al., 2013). Conflict in the early postnatal period increases the likelihood of both parents experiencing depression during the first two years of their child's life (Figueiredo et al., 2017) which, in turn, may lead to poor outcomes for babies and children (El-Sheikh et al., 2009). A father or a mother with a depressed partner may experience a decrease in relationship satisfaction owing to the depressed partner's placing an extra burden on them at a time when they are already coping with the demands of a new baby (Benazon & Coyne, 2000). Individuals with low self-esteem may interpret their partner's responses to the stresses of new parenthood as a negative reflection on their relationship and feel rejected (Don & Mickelson, 2014).

Couple conflict impacts babies' and children's health and wellbeing.

Conflict is also likely to impact the way in which the couple parent their baby, and the extent to which they 'co-parent', that is, engage in consistent behaviours with their baby and responses to their baby's signals that enable the baby to feel secure in terms of his or her needs being met.

Both partners in the relationship, whether same-sex or heterosexual, need to understand the other's response to conflict, and preferred methods of conflict resolution. While research into conflict between *same-sex* couples is limited, studies have shown that conflict between *heterosexual* couples may be fuelled by gender-based differences in communication styles. Women may be more eager to discuss relationship problems than men, whose response to difficulties may be to withdraw from the relationship or pretend that there are no problems (Gottman & Silver, 1999). Men may anticipate that women will be critical of them in discussions about their relationship. This perception may be accurate, as Heyman and colleagues (2009) have reported negativity on the part of women when discussing changes they would like to see in their relationship. Men may therefore find such discussion to be destructive rather than constructive (Ward et al., 2003).

If partners do not share the same ideas about parental roles and responsibilities, marital wellbeing is likely to decrease from pregnancy to the postnatal period (Adamson et al., 2013). The first year of parenthood may also be characterised by a mismatch between expectations of life as new parents and the realities of 24-hour care of a baby. This mismatch may be felt most acutely if the baby is temperamentally demanding, shows negative emotionality and constantly requires parental effort to soothe. In these circumstances, new parents may find that the demands of their newborn overstretch their resources to cope (Oddi et al., 2013).

> The transition to parenthood is a period of adjustment for the mother and the father, but also for the couple.

Belsky and Kelly (1994) argue that couples need to view the transition to parenthood as a period of adjustment for each one individually, but also as a period of adjustment for them as a *couple*. These influential researchers state that couples who see the transition to parenthood as a collaborative experience will work together to meet the challenges that a new baby brings, and thereby reduce each other's stress. If they are able to work as a team, they may well find that their relationship becomes stronger, rather than less satisfying, as they travel through the first weeks and months of new parenting. Pinquart and Teubert (2010) stress the need for early intervention through parent education programmes that target the *couple*.

Into practice

At the turn of this century, a Canadian study (Delmore-Ko et al., 2000) made the following comments and recommendations:

> *Too often, prenatal classes focus only on the birth of the child and then leave the parents to make the actual adjustment to parenthood on their own. Our findings indicate that it would be helpful for expectant parents to discuss postnatal parenting issues prenatally ... It might be beneficial for partners to discuss their expectations about parenthood with one another and become aware of how they differ.*

> (p638)

Early parenting education provides the opportunity for couples to gain in understanding of each other's perspective on new parenthood as well as to acquire knowledge of their baby's needs and development.

Cowan et al. (1985) argue that there are three different experiences of the transition to parenthood: the mother's experience, the father's/partner's experience and the couple's experience. (The baby's experience should also be added!) It is therefore important to offer parenting education in pregnancy and the early postnatal period to *both* parents, and provide couples with opportunities to think *together* about their life with a new baby, rather than engaging only with the mother, leaving her feeling that the major and perhaps sole responsibility for managing the couple's transition to parenthood lies with her.

> Helping pregnant couples develop positive coping strategies together to meet the challenges ahead may prevent decline in relationship satisfaction postnatally.

In recent years, Don and Mickelson (2014) have supported the position that helping pregnant couples develop positive coping strategies to meet the challenges ahead may prevent or diminish decline in relationship satisfaction. Encouraging couples to work together to reflect on and plan for the challenges ahead is a strategy that may protect both parents from poor mental health (Colquhoun & Elkins, 2015). Fostering understanding of each other's feelings about becoming a parent, and building trust and confidence in each one's willingness and ability to support the other, is therefore a key aspect of early parenting education. Houlston et al. (2013) agree, recommending that parent education programmes should target both parenting *and* the couple relationship, with key areas for discussion being:

- Each partner's expectations of the other's role as mother/father
- How the division of household chores might change/should change after the baby is born
- How the couple currently manage conflict in their relationship
- Triggers for conflict that the couple anticipate might occur following the birth of the baby
- Strategies for managing conflict openly and with negotiation.

Educators need to be well trained in order to be able to initiate and shape discussions such as these which are potentially difficult for parents. If the educator is a parent herself (himself), she also needs to have reflected on the way in which having a baby affected her intimate relationship, so that she is free of 'baggage' and able to help couples consider challenges within the context of their very different relationships and personal circumstances.

Listening to each other

For educators to realise the aim of supporting the couple relationship across the transition to parenthood, couples should have plenty of opportunities to share their fears, hopes and ideas both with their peers and with each other. The educator can offer a few minutes of private time in every session for couples to be open about their feelings. Topics for discussion between the couple might be:

- What do you think being a mum/dad is going to be like?
- How hard do you think being a parent is going to be?
- How well do you think you will manage? (The mother should speak for herself, and the father for himself.)

From a basis of insight into each partner's expectations about the transition to parenthood, couples can consider how they will support their relationship. Blinn (2013) suggests an activity for couples to do together where each one completes a series of statements while the other listens without interrupting:

- You support me best when you...
- The greatest strength in our relationship is...
- If I could ask you to change one thing in our relationship, it would be...
- I think that the hardest part of parenting for us will be....
- I think the best part of parenting for us will be... (p24)

Some couples will find such an activity very difficult, and may avoid it by talking about something else. This is their choice. However, many couples will appreciate what may be a rare opportunity to be truly open with each other. Postnatal feedback from one early parenting education programme (Nurturing Parents Preparation for Parenthood Programme, Kirklees, 2015-2016:31) included these comments:

> 'Prompted my partner and I to discuss certain things beforehand that we otherwise wouldn't have.'
>
> 'We had the opportunity in these sessions to discuss how it may affect our relationship. We wouldn't have probably discussed this if it wasn't for these sessions.'

The educator can offer a few minutes of private time in every session for couples to be open about their feelings.

Managing conflict

Early parenting education provides space for pregnant couples to consider relationship challenges at a time when they are open to reflecting on potential difficulties and how to manage them. Problem solving after the baby arrives may be far more difficult. Houts et al. (2008) note that constructive problem solving is most common during the prenatal period, whilst the use of destructive (more harmful) problem solving is highest three months after the birth.

It might be that the only opportunity a couple will ever get to consider how they quarrel and how they could quarrel better will be in an early parenting session. It is another example of how the 'teachable moment of pregnancy' offers the possibility of developing skills and insights that can prove valuable across a lifetime.

A session or part-session on managing conflict might take the following shape.

Opening questions

- What do you think might be the main issues that new parents argue about?
- How do you feel arguing might affect the baby?

Small-group work

Invite the group to break into smaller groups and discuss what keeps relationships positive, and what causes them to become unhappy.

Whole-group work

Introduce the idea that there are different ways in which individuals respond to conflict. Some people become aggressive and attack their partner with angry or humiliating words; some withdraw and refuse to communicate at all; some sulk. Invite the group to share the behaviours they have seen other couples demonstrate.

Video clip

Show a video clip of a couple arguing (an excellent source of such material is the OnePlusOne website: www.oneplusone.org.uk). Ask half of the group to focus on one partner and their way of quarrelling, and the other half to focus on the other partner.

After watching the clip, ask:

- What is driving *x*'s behaviour? How is she feeling?
- What is driving *y*'s behaviour? How is he feeling?
- How is the baby/child feeling?
- How could this argument have been avoided?
- What needs to happen for it to be resolved?
- How can this couple avoid future arguments?
- How can the child/ren be reassured after the argument? How could a baby be reassured?

The following are key messages for parents to take away from a session on managing conflict:

- Conflict is a normal part of relationships
- Making up helps a couple recover from any negative impact of conflict and keeps a relationship strong
- Children benefit from seeing conflict managed well (even babies will sense the 'atmosphere' when parents are quarrelling, and also the change in atmosphere when a disagreement is resolved)
- When conflict is not managed well, children can be harmed in both the short and long term
- The key skills in conflict management are:
  - Recognising when it's time to stop
  - Being able to talk it out
  - Being able to work it out together.

(OnePlusOne 2018, paraphrased)

> Early parenting education may provide the only opportunity a couple will ever get to consider how they quarrel and how they could quarrel better.

Division of labour and prioritising

Prenatally, most couples anticipate equal involvement in childcare and managing the house. However, postnatally, it is most commonly women who assume primary responsibility for these things. Satisfaction with the marital relationship declines when women's prenatal expectations about sharing chores and babycare are not realised (Belsky et al., 1986; Khazan et al., 2008). Therefore, activities and discussions that support couples to understand each other's expectations of who will do what, when and how often after the baby arrives may be helpful.

Couples need time to discuss with each other how to divide household chores postnatally, but it is also helpful to hear how other couples intend to manage. Group discussion may offer couples a different way of thinking about who should do what, and interesting insights into the way in which their priorities match or do not match those of other couples. Therefore, educators might invite the whole group to discuss these issues, and then offer couples time on their own to reflect on the discussion and apply it to their own circumstances.

Couples can be invited to order lists of household tasks and babycare activities according to how important they think each is. Prioritising is a key skill to minimise stress in early parenting. Some couples may consider having a tidy house important; for others, this is irrelevant. Some couples may want to bath their baby daily, and others once a week. In addition, couples need to discuss with each other the importance they attach to pursuing leisure activities, seeing family and friends and going out together. A visit from new parents who can talk about how the priorities they decided on during pregnancy have changed following the birth of their baby may help discussion amongst the pregnant parents to be more realistic and focused.

Conclusion

Novice facilitators may be fearful of providing couples with opportunities to discuss issues that may be difficult for them, or raise awareness of their relationship in a new way. However, Blinn (2013) is encouraging:

> *Initially, I was reluctant to address relationship issues because it seemed to be intruding on a couple's private space. However, over the years, as couples returned to tell their stories to other groups ... I started to see that antenatal*

classes were invaluable in providing the opportunity ... to anticipate the relationship challenges that parenthood brings, and for couples to have discussions with each other about matters which they might otherwise not have broached. One couple who visited my class after their baby had been born told group members that they had learned that the most important thing was 'to be kind to one another' especially when both were so tired and weighed down with the responsibilities of looking after a vulnerable baby. This simple statement clarified for me my responsibility in working with couples during their passage to family life.

(p25)

Key points

Research and theory

- The transition to first-time parenthood has been found to be difficult for many couples
- Conflict between parents impacts children's health and wellbeing
- Conflict impacts the way in which the couple co-parent, and the extent to which they engage in consistent behaviours with their baby and responses to their baby's signals that enable the baby to feel secure
- If partners do not share the same ideas about parental roles and responsibilities, marital wellbeing is likely to decrease from pregnancy to the postnatal period
- Couples who see the transition to parenthood as a collaborative experience work together to meet the challenges that a new baby brings, and thereby reduce each other's stress

Into practice

- It is important to offer early parenting education in pregnancy and the early postnatal period to *both* parents, and therefore provide couples with opportunities to think *together* about their life with a new baby
- Couples need plenty of opportunities to share their fears, hopes and plans with their peers and, in private, with each other
- The educator can support the group to consider how they quarrel and how they could quarrel better
- A visit from new parents who can talk about how they have divided duties in the home and organised their priorities postnatally may help discussion in the antenatal group to be more realistic and focused

Note

In the Appendix are teaching activities, 'Preparing for the realities of early post-natal life', 'Finding time for each other' and 'Managing angry feelings', which may be helpful in facilitating sessions focusing on the couple relationship across the transition to parenthood.

References

Adamson, M., Morawska, A., Sanders, M.R. (2013) Childhood feeding difficulties: A randomized controlled trial of a group-based parenting intervention. *Journal of Developmental and Behavioral Pediatrics*, 34(5):293-302.

Belsky, J., Kelly, J. (1994) *The Transition to Parenthood*. New York: Delacorte.

Belsky, J., Lang, M., Huston, T.L. (1986) Sex typing and division of labor as determinants of marital change across the transition to parenthood. *Journal of Personality and Social Psychology*, 50(3):517-522.

Benazon, N.R., Coyne, J.C. (2000) Living with a depressed spouse. *Journal of Family Psychology*, 14:71-79.

Blinn, M. (2013) Transition to parenting: Balancing the couple's needs and expectations. *International Journal of Birth and Parent Education*, 1(1):23-25.

Colquhoun, G., Elkins, N. (2015) *Healthy Dads? The Challenge of Being a New Father.* Available at: www.beyondblue.org.au/docs/default-source/research-project-files/bw0313-beyondblue-healthy-dads-full-report.pdf?sfvrsn=0 (accessed 11 August 2019).

Cowan, C.P., Cowan, P.A., Heming, G., Coysh, W.S., Curtis-Boles, H. et al. (1985) Transition to parenthood: His, hers and theirs. *Journal of Family Issues*, 6:451-481.

Delmore-Ko, P., Pancer, M.S., Hunsberger, B., Pratt, M. (2000) Becoming a parent: The relation between prenatal expectations and postnatal experience. *Journal of Family Psychology*, 14(4):625-640.

Don, B.P., Mickelson, K.D. (2014) Relationship satisfaction trajectories across the transition to parenthood among low-risk parents. *Journal of Marriage and Family*, 76(3):677-692.

Doss, B.D., Rhoades, G.K., Stanley, S.M., Markman, H.J. (2009) The effect of the transition to parenthood on relationship quality: An 8-year prospective study. *Journal of Personality and Social Psychology*, 96:601-609.

El-Sheikh, M., Kouros, C.D., Erath, S., Cummings, E.M., Keller, P. et al. (2009) Marital conflict and children's externalizing behavior: Interactions between parasympathetic and sympathetic nervous system activity. *Monographs of the Society for Research in Child Development*, 74:vii.

Emery, R.E. (1982) Inter-parental conflict and the children of discord and divorce. *Psychological Bulletin*, 8:160-169.

Feeney, J.A., Hohaus, L., Noller, P., Alexander, R.R. (2001) *Becoming Parents: Exploring the Bonds Between Mothers, Fathers and their Infants*. New York: Cambridge University Press.

Figueiredo, B., Canario, C., Tendais, I., Pinto, T.M., Kenny, D.A. et al. (2017) Couple relationship moderates anxiety and depression trajectories over the transition to parenthood. *European Journal of Public Health*, 27(supplement 3).

Gottman, J.M., Silver, N. (1999) *The Seven Principles for Making Marriage Work*. New York: Three Rivers Press.

Harold, G.T., Congar, R.D. (1997) Marital conflict and adolescent distress: The role of adolescent awareness. *Child Development*, 68:330-350.

Heyman, R.E., Hunt-Martorano, A.N., Malik, J., Slep, A.M.S. (2009) Desired change in couples: Gender differences and effects on communication. *Journal of Family Psychology*, 23:474-484.

Houlston, C., Coleman, L., Mitcheson, J. (2013) Changes for the couple relationship during the transition to parenthood: Risk and protective factors. *International Journal of Birth and Parent Education*, 1(1):18-22.

Houts, R., Barnett-Walker, K.C., Paley, B., Cox, M.J. (2008) Patterns of couple interaction during the transition to parenthood. *Personal Relationships*, 15(1):103-122.

Howard, K.S., Brooks-Gunn, J. (2009) Relationship supportiveness during the transition to parenting among married and unmarried parents. *Parenting, Science and Practice*, 9:123-142.

Huston, T., Holmes, E.K. (2004) Becoming parents. In: Vangelisti, A. (Ed.) *Handbook of Family Communication*. Mahwah, NJ: Erlbaum:105-133.

Khazan, I., McHale, J.P., Decourcey, W. (2008) Violated wishes about division of child-care labor predict early coparenting process during stressful and nonstressful famly evaluations. *Infant Mental Health Journal*, 29(4):343-361.

Lawrence, E., Rothman, A.D., Cobb, R.J., Rothman, M.T. (2008) Marital satisfaction across the transition to parenthood. *Journal of Family Psychology*, 22:41-50.

Nurturing Parents Preparation for Parenthood Programme, Kirklees, 2015-2016. Unpublished report. Available from author.

Oddi, K.B., Murdock, K.W., Vadnais, S., Bridgett, D.J., Gartsein, M.A. (2013) Maternal and infant temperament characteristics as contributors to parenting stress in the first year postpartum. *Infant and Child Development*, 22(6):553-579.

OnePlusOne (2018) *How to Argue Better*. Available at: www.oneplusone.space/how-to-argue-better/ (accessed 21 February 2019).

Perry-Jenkins, M., Goldberg, A.E., Pierce, C.P., Sayer, A.G. (2007) Shift work, role overload and the transition to parenthood. *Journal of Marriage and Family*, 68:123-138.

Petch, J., Halford, W.K. (2008) Psycho-education to enhance couples' transition to parenthood. *Clinical Psychology Review*, 28:1125-1137.

Pinquart, M., Teubert, D. (2010) Effects of parenting education with expectant and new parents: A meta-analysis. *Journal of Family Psychology*, 24(3):316-327.

Towle, C. (1931) The evaluation and management of marital status in foster homes. *American Journal of Orthopsychiatry*, 1:271-284.

Ward, C.A., Bergner, R.M., Kahn, J.H. (2003) Why do men distance? Factors predictive of male avoidance of intimate conflict. *Family Therapy*, 30:1-11.

12 Education and support for same-sex couples

In a mixed group with different family constellations, it is important to make efforts to adjust the content to suit all the families present. Class leaders need to consider the topics they select for group discussion, and how these topics could be adjusted to include all families who may attend their class.

(Malmquist 2016:10)

Research and theory

Research suggests that lesbian women's experience of maternity care is mixed (Lee et al., 2011; Cherguit et al., 2013; Dahl & Malterud, 2015). Some women report favourably on their care, finding that staff treat them with respect; however, others say that staff condescend to them and are clearly prejudiced. This is obviously unacceptable. Same-sex parenting is becoming more common around the world (Gates, 2013) and heterosexual caregivers and educators need to reflect on their attitudes, and evaluate how inclusive the language they use in everyday encounters with pregnant couples is, and whether the care they are providing is non-stigmatising, compassionate and supportive of all couples equally.

Becoming parents presents challenges to the relationship between same-sex couples. Prior to conceiving, a lesbian couple may have had to engage in profound soul searching and make difficult decisions about how to have a baby – who would donate the sperm and who would carry the baby. They have had to think about whether and how the donor should play a part in their child's life.

Research comparing the early parenting experiences of same-sex and heterosexual couples suggests that they face many of the same difficulties (Baiocco et al., 2015). When the baby arrives, gay couples, like heterosexual ones, must cope with tiredness, changes in lifestyle and the weight of responsibility that comes with caring for a new life. Most couples, whatever their sexual orientation, find that they have less time to focus on their own relationship, rather than their relationship with the baby (Goldberg et al., 2014) and that conflict arises more frequently than prior to parenthood. The accumulation of stressors in the first days and months of new parenting threatens all couples' mental and physical health. Depression may be as common in same-sex couples with a new baby as in heterosexual couples (Lavner et al., 2014).

The division of household chores is reported by heterosexual couples to be a focus of conflict in the postnatal period, and articles and books for new parents commonly focus on potential disagreements regarding 'who does what' (e.g. Fisher, 2010). Often, both household chores and essential babycare tasks become gendered in heterosexual relationships after the birth of the baby, in so far as they fall to the at-home parent, generally the mother, while the working father or male partner is less involved. Same-sex couples appear to behave differently and the division of chores remains much the same after the baby's arrival as it was before (Farr & Patterson, 2013).

Research suggests that babies of same-sex couples attach to both parents, and both parents bond equally well with the baby (Goldberg et al., 2012), although there can be problems which do not face heterosexual couples when the birth mother shares a likeness with the baby which identifies the baby as 'hers' rather than her partner's. There is a consensus in the literature that children raised by same-sex parents develop as well emotionally, socially, physically and cognitively as those raised in heterosexual homes (Moore & Stambolis-Ruhstorfer, 2013; Patterson, 2013). Evidence regarding gender-type behaviour of children of same-sex parents suggests either that their play is less gender stereotypical than that of children of heterosexual parents (Goldberg et al., 2012) or that it is no different (Farr et al., 2010).

> Research suggests that babies of same-sex couples attach to both parents, and both parents bond equally well with the baby.

Into practice

Research into what same-sex couples want and need from parent education has focused on lesbian couples; little is known about gay couples. This section, therefore, draws on the (limited) body of evidence about best practice in early parenting education for lesbian couples.

Early parenting education has been found by some lesbian women to be non-inclusive (Larsson & Dykes, 2009). One study (Sabin et al., 2015) found that heterosexual care providers had unconscious antipathy to same-sex couples and preferred to deal with heterosexual couples. A lesbian couple may be the only same-sex couple in a group and educators may fall into the trap of exclusively addressing the normative experiences of a mother, father and baby. The non-birth mother may find herself embarrassed when the antenatal group is divided into 'mothers and fathers', unsure to which group she belongs.

Educators leading early parenting sessions therefore need to become aware of, and then avoid, 'hetero-talk', and reflect on the language they use to ensure it includes lesbian couples. This means that when a lesbian couple are present in the group, it is necessary to avoid the terminology that the educator may commonly employ, that is, referring to the women who are to give birth as 'mothers' and the people who are not going to give birth as 'fathers'. This can be immediately alienating for a lesbian couple and some may not return after the first session. Appropriate language is to refer to the women giving birth as 'mothers' and the other members of the group as 'parents'.

> Educators leading early parenting sessions that include lesbian couples need to become aware of, and then avoid, 'hetero-talk'.

One option for ensuring that lesbian couples feel at ease and free to discuss the particular challenges that they may face is to run early parenting programmes specifically for same-sex couples. In such a setting, couples know that they will not be discriminated against and also that they will not be exposed to the sometimes intrusive and inappropriate questions of heterosexual couples who are keen to know how their baby was conceived and other details of their intimate lives (Malmquist, 2016). Same-sex couples may have concerns about parenting that are not shared by their heterosexual peers. They may fear encountering prejudice at baby groups, at the nursery and the school gates, and be anxious that such prejudice will be directed at their child as well as themselves. Some couples may be coping with hostility from their family members as a result of their choice to have a baby (Gianino, 2008). Early parenting education in a group of same-sex couples allows such concerns to be voiced. Lesbian parents may welcome the opportunity to discuss with other same-sex couples strategies for coping with stigmatisation and discrimination. Such a discussion may be less likely to happen in a group of otherwise heterosexual parents-to-be.

However, there may be insufficient lesbian couples to be able to offer them a dedicated early parenting programme at the appropriate stage of pregnancy. If lesbian couples are to attend general antenatal sessions, educators need to plan beforehand to be sure that every session is inclusive of every parent – giving consideration to the topics covered, how they will be introduced and how discussions about parenting will be shaped. Educators also need to decide whether and how they will split the group into smaller groups. Single-sex small-group work where the intention is to provide a forum for mothers and fathers to have gender-based discussions are likely to be inappropriate. However, couple work is just as important for lesbian as for heterosexual couples and the educator should provide multiple opportunities for partners to talk to each other.

Single-sex small-group work where the intention is to provide a forum for mothers and fathers to have gender-based discussions are likely to be inappropriate in groups which include lesbian couples.

Some topics are of equal importance for educators to address with same-sex as with heterosexual parents. Children's development is strongly affected by the relationship between their parents. If parents support each other in their parenting role, their own mental health is likely to be better and their children less likely to manifest internalising or externalising problems than if there is conflict over parenting approaches (Farr & Patterson, 2013). Early parenting education, therefore, needs to provide opportunities for all couples to consider key issues such as where the baby should sleep, how he or she should be fed and weaned, how often and for how long babies should be exposed to screens and how soon and what kind of bedtime routine to introduce.

As with heterosexual couples, social support has been found to protect the mental health of both parents (Goldberg & Smith, 2011), and therefore, of their child. The importance of early parenting education in enabling same-sex couples to become part of a support group, and of normalising their experiences, cannot be overstated. It is a means of safeguarding the functioning of the new family, and of changing social attitudes. Some same-sex parents will be happy to have a network of largely heterosexual couples for parenting support, but some will look for support primarily to others in their situation and therefore, educators should know where relevant groups are available as well as pointing them in the direction of groups for all parents.

Key points

Research and theory

- Same-sex parenting is becoming more common around the world
- Depression may be as common in same-sex couples with a new baby as in heterosexual couples
- Research suggests that babies of same-sex couples attach to both parents, and the parents bond equally well with the baby

Into practice

- Educators must avoid addressing only the normative experiences of a mother, father and baby
- Educators need to reflect on the language they will use and avoid 'hetero-talk'

- Couple work is as important for lesbian couples as for heterosexual couples
- Single-sex small-group work where the intention is to provide a forum for mothers and fathers to have gender-based discussions may be inappropriate when lesbian parents are attending sessions
- Early parenting education enables same-sex couples to become part of a support group, and normalises their experiences
- Social support protects the mental health of lesbian parents

Note

In the Appendix are teaching activities, 'Preparing for the realities of early post-natal life', 'Finding time for each other' and 'Managing angry feelings', which may be helpful in facilitating sessions focusing on the couple relationship across the transition to parenthood.

References

Baiocco, R., Santamaria, F., Loverno, S., Fontanesi, L., Baumgartner, E. et al. (2015) Lesbian mother families and gay father families in Italy: Family functioning, dyadic satisfaction, and child well-being. *Sexuality Research and Social Policy*, 12:1–11.

Cherguit, J., Burns, J., Pettle, S., Tasker, F. (2013) Lesbian co-mothers' experiences of maternity healthcare services. *Journal of Advanced Nursing*, 69(6):1269–1278.

Dahl, B., Malterud, K. (2015) Neither father nor biological mother: A qualitative study about lesbian co-mothers' maternity care experiences. *Sexual & Reproductive Health Care*, 6(3):169–173.

Farr, R.H., Patterson, C.J. (2013) Coparenting among lesbian, gay and heterosexual couples: Associations with adopted children's outcomes. *Child Development*, 84:1226–1240.

Farr, R.H., Forsell, S.L., Patterson, C.L. (2010) Gay, lesbian and heterosexual parents and their children. *Journal of GLBT Family Studies*, 1:43–61.

Fisher, D. (2010) *Baby's Here! Who Does What? How to Split the Work Without Splitting Up.* Llandovery, Wales: Grandma's Stories.

Gates, G.J. (2013) *LGBT Parenting in the United States* (February). Available at: http://williamsinstitute.law.ucla.edu/wp-content/uploads/LGBT-Parenting.pdf (accessed 30 January 2018).

Gianino, M. (2008) Adaptation and transformation: The transition to adoptive parenthood for gay male couples. *Journal of GLBT Family Studies*, 4:205–243.

Goldberg, A.E., Smith, J.Z. (2011) Stigma, social context, and mental health: Lesbian and gay couples across the transition to adoptive parenthood. *Journal of Counselling Psychology*, 27:431–442.

Goldberg, A.E., Kashy, D.A., Smith, J.Z. (2012) Gender-typed play behaviour in early childhood: Adopted children with lesbian, gay and heterosexual parents. *Sex Roles*, 67:503–515.

Goldberg, A.E., Kinkler, L.A., Moyer, A.M., Weber, E. (2014) Intimate relationship challenges in early parenthood among lesbian, gay and heterosexual couples adopting via the child welfare system. *Professional Psychology: Research and Practice*, 45:221–230.

Larsson, A-K., Dykes, A-K. (2009) Care during pregnancy and childbirth in Sweden: Perspectives of lesbian women. *Midwifery*, 25(6):682–690.

Lavner, J.A., Waterman, J., Peplau, L.A. (2014) Parent adjustment over time in gay, lesbian and heterosexual parent families adopting from foster care. *American Journal of Orthopsychiatry*, 84:46–53.

Lee, E., Taylor, J., Raitt, F. (2011) 'It's not me, it's them': How lesbian women make sense of negative experiences of maternity care – a hermeneutic study. *Journal of Advanced Nursing*, 67(5):982–990.

Malmquist, A. (2016) 'But wait, where should I be, am I Mum or Dad?' Lesbian couples reflect on hetero-normativity in regular antenatal education and the benefits of LGBTQ options. *International Journal of Birth & Parent Education*, 3(3):7–10.

Moore, M.R., Stambolis-Ruhstorfer, M. (2013) LGBT sexuality and families at the start of the twenty-first century. *Annual Review of Sociology*, 39:491–507.

Patterson, C.J. (2013) Children of lesbian and gay parents: Psychology, law and policy. *Orientation and Gender Diversity*, 1(S):27–34.

Sabin, J.A., Riskind, R.G., Nosek, B.A. (2015) Health care providers' implicit and explicit attitudes towards lesbian women and gay men. *American Journal of Public Health*, 105:1831–1841.

13 Education and support for interacting with the baby

Emotional regulation and relationship learning

The architecture of the brain comes to mirror the child's significant experiences.

(Balbernie 2013:26)

Research and theory

The baby's brain grows at a phenomenal pace in the first two years following birth. The person the baby becomes is influenced by his genetic heritage, but the extent to which genes 'express themselves' is determined by his or her earliest experiences:

For the growing brain of a young child, the social world supplies the most important experiences influencing the expression and regulation of genes.

(Siegel 2015:32)

The interactions that the baby has during her first years of life impact the structure of her brain and therefore have long-lasting effects, although neuroscientists are keen to deny that the brain has *no* flexibility after the very early years, but retains the capacity to create new neural networks throughout life (Doidge, 2007). The baby's brain develops in a sequence that gradually but intensively builds her connection with the world around her. Firstly, pathways connected to vision and hearing are established. Language, emotional regulation and higher-level thinking skills come later, but nonetheless have their origins in the first 1000 days.

> The interactions that the baby has during her first years of life impact the structure of her developing brain and therefore have long-lasting effects.

The baby learns about his world through interaction with key caregivers, usually his parents. Emotional and relationship learning is mediated through parents' facial expressions when talking to the baby, through singing, nursery rhymes and music, through reading and holding and stroking. However, the baby's capacity to regulate his emotions is developed primarily through interaction with his parents when he is distressed.

All babies cry – some more than others. This is surely, in part, no more than a reflection of their individuality. Why babies cry is, from an evolutionary perspective, not a difficult question to answer. Human babies are exceptionally vulnerable. They cannot crawl, walk or swim at birth. They have no fur to keep them warm, or even a thick outer layer of skin. If left alone in the wild, they would be a tasty treat for a predator. Babies, therefore, strive to keep themselves safe by ensuring that a more physically developed human being is close to them. They achieve this by 'signalling', that is crying, in order to attract the attention of a caregiver. Babies who are constantly held or carried in a sling close to the mother's body do not cry as much as babies who are regularly put down and left in cots or prams. If the baby is close to an adult, there is no need for him to signal for attention; if he is, as far as he can sense, 'alone', he is bound by thousands of years of human evolution to seek proximity.

During the first two years of life, it is particularly the right side of the brain that is developing – the hemisphere that is affected by and responds to emotions. Whatever needs the baby experiences, she experiences them intensely as her bank of experiences is insufficiently large, and her 'thinking' left brain is insufficiently mature, to enable her to distinguish between 'big' needs and 'little' needs. Once attention from an older human being has been obtained, the baby is then dependent on the caregiver to establish her needs. Crying may be attributed by parents to colic, or discomfort in the digestive tract. Research, however, does not support this idea, even though colic is still commonly referred to by many professionals and parent support groups. The literature suggests that no more than a maximum of 10% of babies have problems with their digestion (Garrison & Christakis, 2000). Tired parents, especially those who are new to parenting, want to find a reason for their baby's crying that is specific and can be remedied by specific treatment. This is why 'colic' is such an attractive explanation – a medical condition that it should be possible to treat with medication or a change in feeding method. However, as Hogg (2015:9) has commented:

> *Parents' focus on trying to treat a stomach problem – for example through increased winding, use of medication and changing bottles and formulas – is likely to be unhelpful for the baby, who may simply need calming, sensitive care.*

Some have argued that a baby who cries 'a lot' (nowhere satisfactorily defined in the literature) is a baby with a difficult temperament who may well find it hard to manage her emotions as she grows up. Once again, there is no foundation in research for such a proposition. It is perhaps more likely that babies who cry a lot are reflecting tensions in the caregiving environment, such as friction between mother and father, or parental anxiety arising from worries about how to care for the baby, or how to keep a roof over her head. Young parents may be especially stressed and unready emotionally and cognitively for parenting, and this may manifest in an unsettled baby (van den Bergh et al., 2009). All of the above, while grounded in common-sense understanding, has not been established in the literature, although many authors have surmised that when parents have limited resources in terms of support or self-efficacy, they are likely to be more worried by, and possibly become more hostile to, their baby's crying (Paulussen-Hoogeboom et al., 2007; Ablow et al., 2013).

> Babies who cry a lot may be reflecting tensions in the caregiving environment.

Common sense might also propose that babies cry when their parents enforce a caregiving regime that does not meet their needs, such as restricting feeds to arbitrary times, and expecting them to settle alone in a room devoid of the smells and sounds of other human beings. This proposal, however, will be disputed by parents who feel that their babies 'conformed' to a strict feeding regime very easily, and settled happily in their own bedroom, away from other members of the family.

Finally, apart from the indisputable logic that human babies require regular contact with a caregiver and are programmed to signal for this if it is not available, there is no overwhelming evidence to support any single cause for what parents might deem 'excessive' crying. Babies cry because they are hungry, because they are wet, or uncomfortable, or over-tired, or hot, or cold, or for any other reason that humans may feel distressed.

Babies and very young children cannot regulate their own emotions. They *feel* strongly, as testified to by a hungry baby's tightly screwed-up face and desperate tearless wails, or a toddler's frantic kicking and screaming when denied the ice-cream on which, as far as he is concerned, his life depends. Indeed, his brain is telling him that his life *does* depend on having the ice-cream because the part of a baby's and young child's brain that is activated in response to perceived need is the primal centre which is focused on survival. It is not for several years, in line with the development of the rational part of the brain, the neocortex, that a child can start to understand and regulate his emotions; for much of childhood, children depend on primary caregivers to manage emotions for them by responding to their signals of distress and enabling the stress hormones that flood their brain when they have a 'need' to be controlled and hormonal harmony restored. It is the way in which the mother and father control the baby's biochemistry by responding or not responding to him that plays a major part in determining whether the future child and adult is able to cope well with stress or feels constantly overwhelmed by life's ups and downs.

> The role of sensitive early parenting is generally recognised by researchers and clinicians to be essential to later emotional regulation.

Children who are confident to draw on external resources (such as a cuddle from mum or dad) to help control their emotions and who develop the capacity to regulate their emotions themselves have been shown to enjoy better relationships with other children and adults, and to have better outcomes at school (Blair & Diamond, 2008). The role of sensitive early parenting is generally recognised by researchers and clinicians to be essential to later emotional regulation (Thompson & Meyer, 2007).

Parenting style is, of course, only one of several factors influencing a child's emotional self-regulation. Each child has a different genetic endowment and temperament, as is evident from the start of life. Some babies are placid and cry only if they are hungry, otherwise appearing content; some seem to have far more labile emotions and their crying can, at times, defeat parents' ability to understand what it is they need. By spending time with their baby, the majority of parents who are not suffering from mental health problems will come to understand how their baby responds to the world he finds himself in, and will become highly skilled in meeting his needs. It is both reassuring and of great significance for early parenting education that research suggests that the impact of stress transmitted from the mother to the baby in pregnancy can be moderated by sensitive postnatal caregiving (Austin et al., 2017).

Into practice

Early parenting education aims to increase parents' understanding of their important responsibility for helping their baby become a child and young person who is not overwhelmed by his emotions but increasingly able to 'roll with the blows' that life deals him.

One of the most important tasks of early parenting is therefore to enable the baby to experience time and time again a sensitive response to whatever emotions he is feeling. The baby thus learns that his emotions can be regulated, that distress can be calmed, and that there is a baseline of security and contentment which he can constantly and reliably return to. His parents create a blueprint for stress regulation which will determine the way in which he manages emotions himself as he grows up.

Crying

The educator can ask group members why babies cry, as they pass a doll from person to person, imagining it to be a crying baby. S/he can then elicit from parents that the overarching reasons for why babies cry are:

- To ensure that he or she maintains contact with a caregiver for protection
- To ensure close physical contact with the mother – an instinctive goal of infants:
    (a) Because babies cannot control their temperature well and need their mother's body warmth to control it for them
    (b) Because, in contrast with other species, human breast milk is low in fat and protein so infants must 'signal' to bring the mother to them so that they can feed regularly to ensure they receive sufficient nutrients.

The group should have an opportunity to discuss whether it is possible to 'spoil' babies by picking them up when they cry. This myth of 'spoiling' is one that people often find very persuasive. The educator needs to explain that a baby's attachment style develops in particular through the parents' response *when the baby is distressed* and that a child who has become securely attached during the first eighteen months of life because he has had his needs met is less likely than insecurely attached children to be clingy at four or five years of age. Contrary to what many people believe, secure attachments tend to foster *autonomy* rather than *dependency*.

In addition, parents deserve to be informed that regularly leaving a baby in the grip of soaring stress hormones harms her immune system, makes it harder for her to learn because the brain's information-processing system is less efficient when under stress and makes her anxious and therefore more vulnerable to poor mental health as she grows up.

The educator can explain to parents that just before and after birth, there is a 'blooming' of brain connections. The baby lays down pathways in her brain that capture what she has learned about how life treats her when she is upset: either that her distress is soothed and therefore she can feel secure in the world, or that her distress is not managed and she is living in a threatening world. At the age of two, nature 'prunes' the pathways that have proliferated in the brain, keeping only the well-used ones. So a child who has been sensitively responded to when distressed keeps the pathways that tell her she is secure and that she can confidently explore her ever-enlarging world. A child whose crying has been ignored in babyhood will have laid down neural pathways that warn her to be cautious in exploring the world as nobody may come to help her if she gets into difficulties.

Secure attachments created during the critical 1000 days foster *autonomy* rather than *dependency*.

Parents may have many questions about this information – and will be fascinated by it. The educator is not aiming to create anxiety and guilt if parents do not always and immediately respond to their baby's crying. She can emphasise that as long as babies' distress is alleviated more often than not, the baby will benefit in terms of becoming increasingly confident to explore and learn as he starts to become mobile and to develop gross and fine motor skills through his first year of life and into his second.

Learning about emotions

A baby needs to learn about the range of emotions that he can experience and what these emotions 'feel' like, 'sound' like and 'look' like. He learns to distinguish between emotions from the way in which his parents reflect his own emotions back to him in the tone of their voice, the way in which they hold him and the expressions on their faces. If the baby is content, he needs to see this reflected in the way his parents become playful with him; if he is upset, he needs to see this mirrored in his parents' concerned facial expressions, the tone of voice they use to talk to him and the close, comforting way they hold him.

Most parents instinctively mirror their baby's emotions. The educator can ask a confident member of the group to hold a doll and react to the 'baby' as if the baby was distressed. And then as if the baby was smiling. Parents will be reassured that they naturally know how to 'teach' their babies about emotions.

Mutual gaze and serve and return

Group members need to understand the importance of interacting with their baby when he is in a receptive state – calm and attentive – rather than always treating such occasions as an opportunity to get on with household chores or other business. The educator can introduce parents to the practice of mutual gaze, when they hold the baby in front of their face and talk to him. This is the earliest kind of interaction which the baby needs:

> Like the serve and return rally in a good game of tennis, young children naturally reach out for interaction with adults through babbling and imitating facial expressions. This process helps them develop important language, cognitive

and social skills. If adults do not respond by getting in sync with children and returning these kinds of noises and gestures, the serve and return rally breaks down and the child's developmental process is interrupted. This has negative implications for later learning.

(Family Support 2019)

Some parents will feel very insecure about communicating with a baby; indeed, the concept may seem bizarre to them. It is helpful for these parents in particular (and for all parents) to learn about 'serve and return' and to witness it in action. Video clips are tremendously useful to show how parents can 'talk' to their baby, listen when the baby 'talks' to them, and then continue the 'conversation'. The educator can point out how the baby manages the conversation with the parent, turning his head away when he needs a rest, and then looking back when he is ready to continue. Parents are fascinated to learn that it is during the 'look-away' moment that the baby's brain consolidates what he is learning from his parent by talking to her, seeing her face and experiencing her touch.

The educator can initiate a discussion about what conditions are necessary for giving attention wholeheartedly to the baby. Parents are likely to mention such strategies as turning their mobile phone and television off, settling down in a comfortable chair with a drink of water or coffee to hand and switching off from thinking about work or household chores.

From the earliest days, parents can talk to their baby about emotions. As language develops fast during the first two years of life, this is the ideal time to help young children build a vocabulary of emotions that will help them later on to express themselves and thereby seek help more effectively when they have problems. As well as naming objects – a vital part of promoting language development – parents can name their emotions. 'I feel really miserable today because I've got a headache'; 'I'm so excited that Auntie JoJo is coming to see us this afternoon'. They can also describe their baby's perceived emotions: 'I think you're grumpy today because you're tired'; 'Are you pleased to see Daddy?' The more the baby and young child hear about emotions, the better is likely to be their understanding of the rich emotional life a human being can experience.

> From the earliest days, parents can talk to their baby about emotions. The more the baby and young child hear about emotions, the better is likely to be their understanding of their emotional life as they grow up.

Interacting through reading

Research (e.g. Niklas & Schneider, 2013) has illuminated the link between book sharing with babies and literacy in later life. The more time adults spend in reading to their babies, the better are likely to be their children's reading skills (Wolf, 2008; Mol & Bus, 2011). However, the primary purpose of reading to babies is not to 'teach' them how to read, but to participate with them in an enjoyable playful interaction. Showing a book to a baby while she is sitting on her parent's knee offers the baby an experience of closeness, warmth, sounds and images that nurture her cognitive and emotional development. The educator can invite parents to list books they remember enjoying at a very early age in their own childhoods, or books that they have read to baby nephews and nieces. Some parents will have had neither of these experiences, and some will find reading difficult. However, Cogan Thacker (2014:16) argues for the importance of *picture* books which provide 'the opportunity for emotional interaction in the earliest book encounters and offer invitations to engage playfully in a language apprenticeship'. For parents with low literacy skills, the emphasis on the importance of *picture* books is reassuring. The message for them and all other parents is that what matters is the 'conversation' that takes place between the parent and baby as the pages are turned and the pictures discussed. Parents may like suggestions to add to their own list of favourites. Cogan Thacker (2014:17) recommends:

- *Each Peach Pear Plum* by Allan and Janet Ahlberg
- *The Very Hungry Caterpillar* by Eric Carle
- *Where's Spot?* by Eric Hill
- *Rosie's Walk* by Pat Hutchins
- *We're Going on a Bear Hunt* by Michael Rosen and Helen Oxenbury
- *The Cat in the Hat* by Dr Seuss
- *The Elephant and the Bad Baby* by Elfida Vipont and Raymond Briggs
- *Goodnight Moon* by Margaret Wise Brown

> Showing a book to a baby while she is sitting on her parent's knee offers the baby an experience of closeness, warmth, sounds and images that nurture her cognitive and emotional development.

Interacting through music

Early parenting education can also touch on the importance of music for young children. Fancourt and Perkins (2017) point to the significant benefits of music for both unborn and newborn babies. The educator can explain to parents that singing to their babies in the womb builds their relationship with him or her and appears to favourably influence neonatal behaviour (Arya et al., 2012) and assist language development (Hallam, 2010). Singing to the baby, or playing music, is a much less expensive, as well as far more effective, way of interacting with the baby than buying a range of educational toys. Mithen (2009) states that being musical is part of our human nature and Patel (2012) explains that the human brain has areas that are especially primed for processing music, and which are linked to other important areas concerned with language development, emotions and movement. It is because sound is so important for babies that human beings all over the world speak to babies in a melodic manner, repeating phrases, using a sing-song lilt and pitching their voices higher than normal. The educator can invite ideas about how to engage the baby musically. Parents may suggest:

- Holding the baby face to face so she can see the parent while s/he is singing
- Bouncing the baby on their knee while singing or reciting nursery rhymes
- Encouraging the slightly older baby to clap to the music
- And the slightly older baby still to 'dance' to music.

The educator can also point out that singing to distressed babies has been shown to be remarkably successful in soothing them (Tafuri, 2009). Some parents will be dismissive of the idea of singing, claiming that they cannot sing – but other parents will point out that babies don't need 'musicians' to interact with them, they need their parents. Henriksson-Macaulay and Welch ((2015:23) note that 'babies are curious and are likely to be open to all types of music'.

Conclusion

While human beings are always able to learn, even if the capacity for and pace of learning diminish in later years, the 1000 days provide a once-in-a-lifetime window of opportunity for diverse and influential learning that will form the basis of how the baby engages with the world of relationships as s/he grows up. From the age of two, the child is still learning frenetically and the brain circuitry is still developing at a considerable rate. However, much learning has already happened and been captured in synaptic connections. Early parenting education must therefore seize the chance to help parents make a positive first impression on their babies' brains because, as Sher (2016) remarks, while there will be opportunities to make a second impression, there is only one opportunity to make a first.

Key points

Research and theory

- The extent to which a baby's genes 'express themselves' is determined by his or her earliest experiences

- During the first two years of life, it is particularly the right side of the baby's brain that is developing - the hemisphere that is affected by and responds to emotions
- Babies strive to keep themselves safe when distressed by 'signalling', that is crying, in order to attract the attention of a caregiver
- Crying may be attributed by parents to colic but research does not support this theory
- The way in which parents respond, or don't respond, to their crying baby plays a major part in determining whether the future child and adult is able to cope well with stress
- The role of sensitive early parenting is generally recognised by researchers and clinicians to be essential to later emotional regulation
- The primary purpose of reading to babies is not to 'teach' them how to read, but to participate with them in an enjoyable playful interaction
- The human brain has areas that are especially primed for processing music, and which are linked to other important areas of the brain to do with language development, emotions and movement

Into practice

- Parents should have an opportunity in early parenting education to discuss whether it is possible to 'spoil' babies by picking them up when they cry
- The educator can introduce parents to the importance of mutual gaze - holding the baby in front of their face and talking to him
- Parents can learn about 'serve and return' through watching a video clip of a parent 'talking' to their baby, listening when the baby 'talks' to them, and then continuing the 'conversation'
- For parents who find reading difficult, the educator can stress the importance of *picture* books for babies as it is the 'conversation' between the parent and baby as the pages are turned, and the pictures discussed, that matters, rather than words on a page
- The educator can inform parents that singing to their baby builds their relationship with her or him and assists language development

Note

In the Appendix are teaching activities, 'Myths and realities about babies' and 'What do you want for your baby? What does your baby need?', which may be helpful in facilitating sessions focusing on interacting with the baby.

References

Ablow, J.C., Marks, A.K., Feldman, S., Huffman, L.C. (2013) Associations between first time expectant women's representations of attachment and their physiological reactivity to infant cry. *Child Development*, 844:1373–1391.

Arya, R., Chansoria, M., Konanki, R., Tiwari, D.K. (2012) Maternal music exposure during pregnancy influences neonatal behaviour: An open-label randomized controlled trial. *International Journal of Pediatrics*, doi.org/10.1155/2012/901812.

Austin, M.P., Christl, B., McMahon, C., Kildea, S., Reilly, N. et al. (2017) Moderating effects of maternal emotional availability on language and cognitive development in toddlers of mothers exposed to a natural disaster in pregnancy: The QF2011 Queensland Flood Study. *Infant Behavior and Development*, 49:296–309.

Balbernie, R. (2013) Poised to connect: How early relationships affect brain development. *International Journal of Birth and Parent Education*, 1(1):26–28.

Blair, C., Diamond, A. (2008) Biological processes in prevention and intervention: The promotion of self-regulation as a means of preventing school failure. *Development and Psychopathology*, 20(3):899–911.

Cogan Thacker, D. (2014) Playing with the text: The importance of sharing books with babies. *International Journal of Birth and Parent Education*, 2(1):15–17.

Doidge, N. (2007) *The Brain that Changes Itself*. London: Penguin Books.

Family Support (2019) Brain development metaphors. Available at: www.family-support.org. uk/who-we-are/brain-development-metaphors (accessed 13 March 2019).

Fancourt, D., Perkins, R. (2017) Maternal engagement with music up to nine months post-birth: Findings from a cross-sectional study in England. *Psychology of Music*, 46(2):238–251.

Garrison, M.M., Christakis, D.A. (2000) A systematic review of treatments for infant colic. *Paediatrics*, 106(1):184–190.

Hallam, S. (2010) The power of music: Its impact on the intellectual, social and personal development of children and young people. *International Journal of Music Education*, 28(3):269–289.

Henriksson-Macaulay, L., Welch, G.F. (2015) The musical key to babies' cognitive and social development. *International Journal of Birth and Parent Education*, 2(2):21–25.

Hogg, S. (2015) Understanding and responding to excessive crying. *International Journal of Birth and Parent Education*, 2(4):7–11.

Mithen, S. (2009) The music instinct: The evolutionary basis of musicality. *Annals of the New York Academy of Sciences*, 1169:3–12.

Mol, S.E., Bus, A.G. (2011) To read or not to read: A meta-analysis of print exposure from infancy to early adulthood. *Psychological Bulletin*, 137(2):267–296.

Niklas, F., Schneider, W. (2013) Home literacy environment and the beginning of reading and spelling. *Contemporary Educational Psychology*, 38:40–50.

Patel, A.D. (2012) Language, music and the brain: A resource-sharing framework. In: Rebuschat, P., Rohmeier, P., Hawkins, M., Cross, I. (Eds.) *Language and Music as Cognitive Systems*. Oxford: Oxford University Press: 204–223.

Paulussen-Hoogeboom, M.C., Stams, G.J., Hermanns, J.M., Peetsma, T.T. (2007) Child negative emotionality and parenting from infancy to preschool: A meta-analytic review. *Developmental Psychology*, 43(2):438–453.

Sher, J. (2016) *Missed Periods: A Primer on Preconception Health, Education and Care*. An independent report commissioned by NHS Greater Glasgow and Clyde (Public Health). Available at: www.drugsandalcohol.ie/26068/1/missed-periods-Scotand_pregnancies. pdf (accessed 23 November 2019).

Siegel, D.J. (2015) *The Developing Mind: How Relationships and the Brain Interact to Shape Who We Are (2nd Ed.)*. New York: Guilford Press.

Tafuri, J. (2009) *Infant Musicality: New Research for Educators and Parents*. Translated by Elizabeth Hawkins and edited by Graham Welch. Farnham: Ashgate.

Thompson, R.A., Meyer, S. (2007) Socialization of emotion regulation in the family. In: Gross, J.J. (Ed.) *Handbook of Emotion Regulation.* New York: Guilford Press: 249-268.
Van den Bergh, M.P., van der Ende, J., Crijnen, A.A., Jaddoe, V.W., Moll, H.A. et al. (2009) Paternal depressive symptoms during pregnancy are related to excessive infant crying. *Pediatrics,* e98-e104.
Wolf, M. (2008) *Proust and the Squid.* Cambridge: Icon Books.

14 Education and support for breastfeeding

Breastfeeding is a natural 'safety net' against the worst effects of poverty ... Exclusive breastfeeding goes a long way toward cancelling out the health difference between being born into poverty and being born into affluence ... It is almost as if breastfeeding takes the infant out of poverty for those first few months in order to give the child a fairer start in life and compensate for the injustice of the world into which it was born.

(James P. Grant, former Executive Director of UNICEF)

Research and theory

Human milk is perfectly adapted to the needs of human babies. This is a statement that is often made by health professionals to persuade mothers and families that breastfeeding offers their babies the best possible start in life. Perhaps the statement has been made so often that it has lost its impact. And there are authoritative voices telling parents that:

Breastfeeding is not the panacea some might think. There is data to support that nursing improves the short-term health of your baby in a few specific ways (fewer allergic rashes, intestinal disorders and ear infections), but the data is not there on its long-term benefits (breastfed kids are not smarter, or necessarily have lower risks of obesity, cancer, diabetes).

(Emily Oyster, Professor of Economics, Brown University, USA, speaking on BBC *Woman's Hour*, 18 July 2019)

Such extraordinarily misleading and partial statements, which are clearly set in a Western context (Oyster fails to register that breastfeeding ensures the *survival* of many babies in countries where there is an inadequate and polluted water supply) and which take no account of the benefits of breastfeeding for the *mother* or of its role in terms of bonding and attachment, may, however, be used as justification by parents for not breastfeeding or for stopping earlier than the six months recommended by the World Health Organization (2011).

Educators now have to challenge themselves to present the facts about breastfeeding in a way that stimulates parents' enthusiasm for the amazing qualities of breast milk and the special closeness that breastfeeding enables the mother and baby to enjoy.

Whatever the environmental conditions prevalent when a human baby is born, the mother is able to synthesise milk that meets the baby's requirements in those circumstances. The baby is therefore not dependent on the mother's having access to a variety of food or even enough food. The mother may suffer from hunger or an unbalanced diet but the baby can still receive all the nutrients he needs for survival and healthy development from her milk.

However, unlike other mammals, human milk must be delivered to the baby at very regular intervals:

> *As mammals, human infants have evolved to be breastfed. They have evolved the biological expectation that they will be in proximity with a caregiver at all times, and that they will breastfeed frequently throughout the day and night.*
>
> (Rudzik 2018:10)

While some animals feed their offspring milk that is rich in carbohydrates and protein to enable their infants to remain satisfied for long periods of time while the mother leaves them to look for food, others, including the human animal, feed their babies a milk that is low in carbohydrate and protein, but high in lactose. This is milk suitable for infants who are *carried* by their mothers from place to place, not left alone in a burrow or nest. Breastfeeding therefore necessitates mothers staying close to their infants.

It is a commonly held belief that breastfeeding mothers get less sleep during the night than bottle-feeding mothers because their babies wake more frequently. In fact, Rudzik et al. (2018) found that there was no difference between the sleep times of breastfed and bottle-fed babies. A seminal study (Galland et al., 2012) of sleep patterns amongst infants during the first two years of life concluded that there is great variability from baby to baby in terms of the number of night wakings and the overall length of time they spend asleep, with night waking being commonplace in the first months of life right through to two years of age.

A review of studies comparing breastfeeding education delivered by health professionals either to women individually, or in groups, concludes (as is so often the case with studies of early parenting education) that:

> *The methodological heterogeneity and the small number of high quality studies limited our ability to draw firm conclusions about the effectiveness of either mode of antenatal education.*
>
> (Wong et al. 2015)

However, this study comments on the effectiveness of any form of breastfeeding education for women least likely to initiate it – those from low-income, low-education and minority families. Breastfeeding education targeted at these groups has some positive impact on the length of exclusive breastfeeding, or any breastfeeding, *provided that* educators have the skills to be able to tailor their sessions to overcome barriers of language, learning style and possible hostility arising from a previous history of unfulfilling and unenjoyable education.

> Skilled breastfeeding education, whether in groups or for individuals, has been shown to have a positive impact on the women least likely to initiate it – those from a low-income, low-education background, and/or from minority families.

The language that has been used to promote breastfeeding has often proved problematic. Mothers participating in the study by Brown (2016) commented that the 'breast is best' message had two unintended implications: firstly, it suggests that, while formula feeding might not be 'best', it is good enough; and, secondly, it implies that breastfeeding requires unusual expertise as achieving what is 'best' in life usually involves extensive practice to fine-tune complex skills.

Brown (2016) advocates describing breastfeeding as the 'normal' way to feed a baby; *nature* chooses breastfeeding for human babies. Formula feeding then becomes a choice made by *parents*. Referring to breastfeeding as normal (even if not the *usual* way to feed a baby in many contemporary societies) and formula feeding as a *different* form of nurturance is to describe the two ways of feeding a baby accurately.

Into practice

While there is no consensus regarding the most effective way in which to deliver prenatal breastfeeding education (Wong et al., 2015), providing it in a hospital or clinical setting, as is often the case, may not be ideal. Doing so risks conveying the message that breastfeeding is 'a medical matter', may well require medical intervention and is not a normal, everyday human behaviour.

Educators need to be clear when constructing a breastfeeding session that a single session delivered in pregnancy will not be sufficient to ensure, or even make it more likely, that the women attending will initiate and sustain exclusive, or even some, breastfeeding. Prenatal input has to be backed up with further education in the postnatal period, delivered either in groups or one to one, and with support at breastfeeding 'cafes' and in groups run by volunteers from the variety of charities with a mission to promote breastfeeding and support new families. Imdad et al. (2011) note that professional support can be enhanced by support and education provided by lay people, and that this leads to increased exclusive breastfeeding at four to six weeks and at six months. De Oliveira et al. (2001) state that breastfeeding education and support should be offered *across the transition to parenthood*, both during pregnancy and after the baby is born. The review by Wong et al. (2015) makes the same point.

Therefore, a key element of the antenatal session must be signposting women and their families to these later educational and support opportunities. Every participant in a prenatal early parenting session needs to leave with a leaflet listing the local breastfeeding support groups and baby cafes, with up-to-date times and venue details, and also the contact numbers (again, regularly updated by the educator) for breastfeeding counsellors and links to reliable breastfeeding websites. Perhaps the most important message to be conveyed in prenatal breastfeeding sessions is that women and their partners and families *are not alone* once they start their breastfeeding journey.

> The most important message to be conveyed in prenatal breastfeeding sessions is that women and their partners and families *are not alone* once they start their breastfeeding journey.

Avoiding coercion

The large survey undertaken by Brown (2016) showed that, despite highly publicised controversies on social media about perceived over-zealous promotion of breastfeeding by health professionals, mothers were very much in favour of breastfeeding education. However, they did not want to feel coerced. Some participants at a parenting education session on breastfeeding will be very committed to this method of feeding their baby; others will have come along out of interest or because they feel they 'should' learn more about breastfeeding even though their preference is to formula feed. Any hint of coercion is likely to alienate these latter groups. The 'breast is best' message has overplayed its hand. Women have made it clear on social media that they dislike feeling bullied or shamed into breastfeeding, castigating those whom they see as 'nipple Nazis' and 'breastfeeding mafia'.

> Women don't like:
>
> The 'message' that breastfeeding is the only way to feed a baby.

> An exclusive focus on breastfeeding rather than on infant feeding.
> A lack of information about bottle feeding.
>
> (Nurturing Parents Preparation for Parenthood
> Programme, Kirklees 2015-2016:29)

Making it clear at the start of a session on infant feeding that this is an opportunity for parents to air their views on how best to feed their babies, and to hear other people's ideas, and that all viewpoints are welcome and will be respected, emphasises that the session is not intent on coercing parents to make 'the right decision' about infant feeding. Educators can make a clear statement that their aim is to help every woman/couple make the decision that feels best for them, and to carry out that decision safely and happily. Educators protect themselves from accusations of bias by asking parents what information they want, and then eliciting that information, as far as possible, from the group itself. When information is provided by parents and supplemented by the educator, parents are likely to feel ownership of the session.

Educators need to be very aware of the risk of their own position on breastfeeding affecting the way in which they shape the session and respond to parents' views. Almost certainly, one or several parents will present the argument that many babies seem to thrive on formula milk, and develop into happy and healthy toddlers. This observation may weigh heavily with parents who are doubtful about the superiority of breastfeeding. It can be difficult to 'manage' such a discussion when the educator feels strongly and perhaps even passionately that every baby should be breastfed, and understands the evidence that toddlers who appear to be as healthy as their breastfed sisters and brothers may, in fact, not be so. This is an occasion where the educator needs to sit back and allow the group to debate the issue; almost certainly, there will be well-informed parents present who will make the points that the educator her- or himself would have made. The fact that it is parents making them will be far more influential with the rest of the group than if they had come from the educator. There may, of course, be opportunity for the educator to share some facts that group members are unaware of, but trying to monopolise the discussion in order to steer it in the 'right' direction will not persuade undecided parents.

An opening activity that may draw out feelings about infant feeding could be to display a range of pictures of babies being breast- and bottle-fed and then invite group members to choose one that they like or dislike and say why. If this activity goes well, it may be that the rest of the session can be built on it. For example, a mother may comment that she likes a picture illustrating how the baby is so close to the mother while breastfeeding. Another may say that she has chosen a picture of a mother bottle feeding because she thinks bottle feeding will be easier and that breastfeeding would hurt. A father may say that the breastfeeding pictures make him feel left out, and that as feeding the baby is such a special thing, he would like to be part of it, too. Drawing on these comments, the educator might develop parents' ideas in the following ways:

- Feeding isn't just about putting milk into a baby. It's also about closeness. We've talked previously about why closeness, such as with skin to skin, is so important for the development of the baby. Mother and baby have to be close if the baby is breastfeeding. However, closeness can also be part of bottle feeding – have you any thoughts about this?
- Breastfeeding problems are nearly all related to how the baby is attached to the breast. Has anyone seen a baby breastfeed? What does it look like? (From the information offered, the educator can move on to look at correct positioning at the breast and offer dolls to couples who want to practise, so that they can appreciate that breastfeeding doesn't mean holding the baby in the crook of the arm, but letting the baby face the breast so he doesn't have to twist his neck to feed. A video of correct attachment may be helpful.)
- Do fathers and partners feel that breastfeeding excludes you from having a special relationship with your baby? What have friends said to you about this? How can you ensure that you're part of breastfeeding, and that you develop your own unique relationship with your baby?

Involving key family members

Wouk et al. (2016) are clear that:

> Prenatal interventions have been found to be effective in increasing breastfeeding initiation, duration and exclusivity, where they combine edu- cation with interpersonal support and <u>where they involve women's partners or family</u>.
>
> (p51) (author's underlining)

The effectiveness of including women's husbands, partners and significant family members in breastfeeding education receives considerable support from a raft of studies conducted in the last fifteen years (e.g. Maycock et al., 2013; Bich et al., 2014; Bonuck et al., 2014). Yet research findings have not been translated universally, or even extensively, into practice, with many women attending 'the breastfeeding class' during the day when their partners are unable to come with them.

Brown and Davies (2014) identify the significant challenge for breastfeeding education in ensuring that information is directed equally at fathers as well as at prenatal and postnatal mothers. In their study, men reported 'being excluded from antenatal breastfeeding education or being considered unimportant in postnatal support' (p510). Yet fathers play a significant role in breastfeeding

(Everett et al., 2006; Tohotoa et al., 2009; Sherriff & Hall, 2011). Without the support of fathers/partners, women are far more likely to change to formula feeding if difficulties with breastfeeding arise. The attitudes of grandmothers and other female relatives of the mother may also be very significant (Rollins et al., 2016). Breastfeeding is not the sole responsibility of the mother; supporting breastfeeding is a family responsibility, and the responsibility of the wider community as well.

> It is vital to ensure that breastfeeding information is directed equally at fathers and partners as well as at prenatal and postnatal mothers.

It is vital that fathers/partners are included in all early parenting sessions on infant feeding, and respected as equally important as the mother, both in the infant feeding decision and in its management. Men want *specific* information about breastfeeding; too 'lyrical' an account of its benefits may not satisfy them. For example, they may find a comparison of the nutrients available in breast milk and those in formula milk very compelling. They may appreciate being shown how much money breastfeeding can save, and welcome an explanation of why 'stretching' formula milk to make it go further, thereby cutting the cost of buying it, is highly detrimental to babies' health. Educators might, therefore, initiate an activity based on a document such as the First Steps Nutrition Trust's report on the *Cost of Infant Milks Marketed in the UK* (2018) and ask group members to work out how much formula feeding a baby for the first year of life might cost.

Fathers are often concerned about the disruption to night-time sleep occasioned by breastfeeding. Educators can discuss the research that shows that breast- and bottle-feeding mothers have been found to get roughly the same amount of sleep in the first year of their baby's life. If both groups of babies are fed on demand, and parents choose not to use 'sleep extinction' strategies such as 'cry it out' and 'controlled crying', bottle-fed and breastfed babies develop similar sleeping patterns as they move towards the second year of life (Rudzik et al., 2018).

Father-focused factsheets to take home are likely to be appreciated.

Breastfeeding for men

- *Breastfeeding represents an incredible opportunity for the human brain (and the body, in general) to reach its full potential*

- *Breast milk is a natural, renewable food that is environmentally safe and produced and delivered to the baby without pollution, unnecessary packaging or waste*
- *Formula milk needs energy to manufacture, materials for packaging, fuel for transport and water, fuel and cleaning agents for daily preparation and use*
- *Women who have a partner who is informed, supportive and encouraging are more likely to start breastfeeding and breastfeed for longer*
- *The first few days after birth are important for getting the baby to attach to the breast comfortably and for the mother to find the best feeding positions for her. Newborn babies want to feed often in the first weeks. This is important as it will help to establish an adequate milk supply and the time between feeds will settle over the next few months*
- *Help your partner find a comfortable position for feeding. Leaning back as if lying in a deckchair, with the baby supported by her body, is a good position. But whatever works for her and the baby is great*
- *Breastfeeding is thirsty work for mother and baby. A healthy diet and plenty of water are important. Offer her snacks while she's feeding, such as fruit, yoghurt, hard-boiled eggs and crackers with cheese or Marmite*
- *Get help, if you need it, earlier rather than later. Midwives, health visitors, public health nurses, lactation consultants and breastfeeding counsellors are available to help you. You can also ring helplines run by charities, such as the NCT Breastfeeding Helpline and the Association of Breastfeeding Mothers*
- *Conflicting advice can be a problem. Find one person or organisation that you trust and stick with them*
- *Ask for help for yourself if you're finding it difficult to help your partner*

Fathers/partners also want information about how they can support the mother practically. The educator can set up single-sex small groups and invite mothers to think about what help they want from their partners with breastfeeding, and fathers/partners to consider what they can offer. Both groups may welcome the opportunity to discuss their feelings away from their partners and receive confirmation from, or be challenged by, their peer group. At the end of the time available for discussion, each group can be invited to offer their thoughts to the other. This discussion should be followed by a couple of minutes for each couple to talk together about how they will *both* be involved in feeding their baby.

Realistic preparation

It is vital to prepare women and men *realistically* for breastfeeding. There may be a temptation on the part of educators to try to 'sell' breastfeeding by focusing on its undisputed health benefits to the point that parents see it as a pass to perfect health, leaving them feeling disappointed and cheated when their breastfed baby *does* suffer from the common coughs, colds and sticky eyes of the first year of life. It is dishonest to paint a picture of breastfeeding that does not include a realistic portrayal of the likely challenges that couples will face. Telling stories about breastfeeding is as important as telling stories about labour and birth. Inviting breastfeeding counsellors and parents with a young baby to talk about the ups and downs of breastfeeding will enrich antenatal breastfeeding education:

> *I went to this great class. We covered why breastfeeding is so important and how to do it but also what it was really like to breastfeed. Some local peer supporters came in and fed in front of us (which was the first time I had seen a baby breastfeed) and talked about problems they had and importantly how they got over them. They then gave us details of how to contact them and groups to go to once the baby was here. We felt part of something and like we knew what to expect.*
>
> (quote from mother in study by Brown 2016:106)

While there are many advantages to exclusive breastfeeding and it is the *normal* way to feed a young human being, there are many pressures operating on new parents in Western societies that make exclusive breastfeeding difficult to maintain. Many couples will, in the early weeks of their baby's life, make the decision to introduce formula as a supplement to, or instead of, breastfeeding. It is important that they shouldn't feel 'guilty' about their decision. The educator's aim is to encourage *any* breastfeeding and the message to parents is that even one day of breastfeeding is good for the baby. Six months of exclusive breastfeeding as advocated by the World Health Organization (2011) is excellent for mothers and babies, but *every* breastfeed is a positive act. The educator aims to encourage mothers and couples to take 'one day at a time'.

Important in terms of presenting breastfeeding realistically (and infant feeding in general) is to help couples appreciate the number of times a baby needs to feed every day and the irregularity of feeds. A simple activity such as inviting each couple to fill in a 24-hour timeline for their new baby, imagining what his or her sleep/wake times might be, and charting periods when the baby might be unsettled can help highlight the unpredictability of infant feeding in the first months of life. Each couple's timeline will be different. The educator can then lay out seven of the timelines randomly, one for each day of the week, and explain that in the first week, the baby may feed and sleep from day to day as illustrated by the seven timelines; but in the second week, may feed in a pattern illustrated by a completely different way of arranging the timelines. The educator can explain that a baby may sometimes go quite long periods between feeds, sometimes cluster feed and often want to feed at least as much during the night as in the day. The aim of this activity is therefore to raise parents' awareness of the unpredictability of very young babies' days, and to buffer their mental health by helping them develop realistic expectations of early parenting. Visual aids illustrating how small a newborn baby's tummy is and, therefore, how regularly it will need filling if the baby is to double his or her birth weight by six months, as is usual, are highly persuasive and fascinating to parents.

Breastfeeding stories meet the need for realistic preparation for the post-natal period.

Avoiding information overload

In constructing a prenatal breastfeeding session, educators need to decide how much can reasonably be covered in the time available bearing in mind that information overload is counter-productive, the kind of information that is most useful for group members to have *while they are pregnant*, and what information and skills should be kept for further education in the postnatal period. The content of the session/s will be shaped by each educator's experience of what kind of breastfeeding education is helpful during pregnancy, by the requirements of the institution for which s/he is working and, of course, by what parents ask to be told about. In the study by Brown and Davies (2014), fathers particularly wanted to know about problems that could arise with breastfeeding, and how to tackle them. It may be appropriate, therefore, to invite group members to share difficulties that friends or relatives have experienced and to look briefly at the source of these problems (nearly always incorrect positioning) and the way in which mothers and fathers/partners might respond to them. A useful topic for discussion is whether it is a good idea for breastfeeding parents to have bottles and formula in the house 'just in case' breastfeeding proves challenging. Educators need to be skilled to ensure that the entire session is not hijacked by parents fretting over 'things going wrong' and 'horror stories' about other parents' experiences. Pregnancy is an opportunity primarily for signposting in relation to breastfeeding. Most parents will be satisfied if given some literature about common breastfeeding problems, or directed to quality websites, and reminded that if problems arise – and there is no certainty that they will – there are people who can help them.

There are other topics that parents may wish to discuss or that educators feel important to introduce, for example, whether and how to breastfeed in public places. Despite all four governments in the UK supporting breastfeeding, including in public, many women are surprisingly shy about exposing their breasts even though breasts are on display in every magazine, TV advert, billboard and shop window. Fathers/partners may have strong feelings about breastfeeding in public and these need sharing in the group and ways of breastfeeding discreetly demonstrated.

A breastfeeding session might be brought to a close with a renewed emphasis on seeking help before problems become serious. As well as offering information on the availability of breastfeeding support sessions, the educator may also be able to offer a text messaging service as an inexpensive and effective means of reinforcing key messages, and of advising and supporting parents in the first weeks after their baby is born (Gallegos et al., 2014).

Key points

Research and theory

- Whatever the environmental conditions prevalent when a human baby is born, the mother is able to synthesise milk that meets the baby's requirements in those circumstances
- Unlike the milk of some other mammals, human milk must be delivered to the baby at very regular intervals
- Research has found that there is no difference between the amount of time breastfed and bottle-fed babies spend asleep
- *Every* breastfeed is a positive act
- Without the support of fathers/partners, women are far more likely to change to formula feeding if difficulties with breastfeeding arise

Into practice

- Educators need to be aware of their own position regarding breastfeeding in order to avoid coercion in the way they lead a breastfeeding session and respond to parents' views
- Educators have to meet the challenge of presenting the facts about breastfeeding in a new light and re-awakening parents' enthusiasm for the amazing qualities of breast milk and the special closeness that breastfeeding enables the mother and baby to enjoy
- A single breastfeeding education session delivered in pregnancy will not be sufficient to ensure that women initiate and sustain breastfeeding. Antenatal input has to be backed up with further education postnatally
- Educators need to decide how much information can reasonably be offered in the time available and what it is useful for parents to know

while *they are pregnant*, and what should be kept for further education in the postnatal period

- Referring to breastfeeding as *normal* (even if it is not the *usual* way to feed a baby in our society) and formula feeding as a *different* form of nurturance is an accurate way to describe infant feeding choices
- Educators need to make clear at the start of the session that everyone's views on how to feed a baby will be welcome and respected
- It is essential to include women's husbands, partners and significant family members in breastfeeding education
- Information should be directed equally at fathers/partners as well as at mothers
- Fathers/partners want to know how they can *practically* support the mother
- Sharing stories about breastfeeding is an important means of providing a realistic account of what is involved
- A key element of an antenatal breastfeeding session is signposting women and their families to support groups and further educational opportunities

Note

In the Appendix are teaching activities, 'Myths and realities about babies' and 'Feeding stars', which may be helpful in facilitating sessions focusing on early infant care and feeding.

References

Bich, T.H., Hoa, D.T.P., Målqvist, M. (2014) Fathers as supporters for improved exclusive breastfeeding in Viet Nam. *Maternal and Child Health Journal*, 18:1444-1453.

Bonuck, K., Stuebe, A., Barnett, J., Labbok, M.H., Fletcher, J. et al. (2014) Effect of primary care intervention on breastfeeding duration and intensity. *American Journal of Public Health*, 104 (Suppl.1):S119-S127.

Brown, A. (2016) What do women really want? Lessons for breastfeeding promotion and education. *Breastfeeding Medicine*, 11(3):102-110.

Brown, A., Davies, R. (2014) Fathers' experiences of supporting breastfeeding: Challenges for breastfeeding promotion and education. *Maternal & Child Nutrition*, 10:510-526.

de Oliveira, M.I., Camacho, L.A., Tedstone, A.E. (2001) Extending breastfeeding duration through primary care: A systematic review of prenatal and postnatal interventions. *Journal of Human Lactation*, 17(4):326-343.

Everett, K.D., Bullock, L., Gage, J.D., Longo, D.R., Geden, E. et al. (2006) Health risk behaviour of rural low-income fathers. *Public Health Nursing*, 23(4):297-306.

First Steps Nutrition Trust (2018) Cost of infant milks marketed in the UK (2018). Available at: https://static1.squarespace.com/static/59f75004f09ca48694070f3b/t/5afc61278a922d5d7ff9da5a/1526489384704/Costs_of_Infant_Milks_Marketed+_in_the_UK_May_2018.pdf (accessed 24 Novembe 2019).

Galland, B.C., Taylor, B.J., Elder, D.E., Herbison, P. (2012) Normal sleep patterns in infants and children: A systematic review of observational studies. *Sleep Medicine Reviews*, 16(3):213–222.

Gallegos, D., Russell-Bennett, R., Previte, J., Parkinson, J. (2014) Can a text message a week improve breastfeeding? *BMC Pregnancy and Childbirth*, 14:374.

Imdad, A., Yakoob, M.Y., Bhutta, Z.A. (2011) Effect of breastfeeding promotion interventions on breastfeeding rates with special focus on developing countries. *BMC Public Health*, 11 (Suppl. 3):S24.

Maycock, B., Binns, C.W., Dhaliwal, S., Tohotoa, J., Hauck, Y. et al. (2013) Education and support for fathers improves breastfeeding rates: A randomized controlled trial. *Journal of Human Lactation*, 29(4):484–490.

Nurturing Parents Preparation for Parenthood Programme, Kirklees, 2015–2016. Unpublished report. Available from author.

Rollins, N.C., Bhandari, N., Hajeebhoy, N., Horton, S., Lutter, C.K. et al. (2016) Why invest, and what will it take to improve breastfeeding practices? *The Lancet*, 387(10017):491–504.

Rudzik, A. (2018) Infant sleep and feeding in evolutionary perspective. *International Journal of Birth and Parent Education*, 6(1):9–12.

Rudzik, A.E.F., Robinson-Smith, L., Ball, H.L. (2018) Discrepancies in maternal reports of infant sleep vs actigraphy by mode of feeding. *Sleep Medicine*, 49:90–98.

Sherriff, N., Hall, V. (2011) Engaging and supporting fathers to promote breastfeeding: A new role for health visitors? *Scandinavian Journal of Caring Sciences*, 25:467–475.

Tohotoa, J., Maycock, B., Hauck, Y.L., Howat, P., Burns, S. et al. (2009) Dads make a difference: An exploratory study of paternal support for breastfeeding in Perth, Western Australia. *International Breastfeeding Journal*, 4(15). Available at: https://international breastfeedingjournal.biomedcentral.com/track/pdf/10.1186/1746-4358-4-15?site=intern ationalbreastfeedingjournal.biomedcentral.com (accessed 1 January 2018).

Wong, K.L., Tarrant, M., Lok, K.Y.W. (2015) Group versus individual professional antenatal breastfeeding education for extending breastfeeding duration and exclusivity: A systematic review. *Journal of Human Lactation*, 31(3):354–366.

World Health Organization (WHO) (2011) Exclusive breastfeeding for six months best for babies everywhere. Available at: www.who.int/mediacentre/news/statements/2011/ breastfeeding_20110115/en/ (accessed 26 February 2019).

Wouk, K., Tully, K.P., Labbok, M. (2016) Systematic review of evidence for Baby-Friendly Hospital Initiative Step 3: Prenatal breastfeeding education. *Journal of Human Lactation*, 33(1):50–82.

15 Education and support for young mothers

Many of the young women felt proud about the ways in which they were bringing up their children and felt positive about being a mother: 'It's great, I love it. She's really good, she hasn't got any teeth yet but she's doing all the other things, crawling, pulling herself up the stairs, trying to walk' ... Tina, 16 years old, with 9-month-old daughter.

(McDermott & Graham 2005:70)

Research and theory

The UK under-eighteen conception rate in 2016 was 18.9 conceptions per thousand women aged fifteen to seventeen years – the lowest rate recorded since comparable statistics were introduced in 1969 (Office for National Statistics (ONS), 2018).This reduction may be considered cause for celebration as it is known that babies of teenage mothers are at increased risk of low birthweight, of being stillborn, of dying in infancy and of not being breastfed, while their mothers are more likely than older ones not to be in education, employment or training (Public Health England, 2016). Many young mothers are living in poverty; many are care-leavers who have experienced little or no continuity of loving, sensitive parenting in their own childhoods, and many have experienced physical and emotional abuse (Swann et al., 2002).

Yet it is easy to fall into the trap of viewing every teenage pregnancy as some kind of disaster when, in many parts of the world, it would be the norm. Every young woman who comes to an early parenting course will have a different story to tell (although they may not tell it) about the circumstances under which they became pregnant and, more importantly, why. Some are pregnant because it is customary in their culture, or their families, to bear children at an early age – many of these young women will have good support systems around them to ease their pathway into parenthood. Other teenagers have deliberately chosen to get pregnant, seeing parenthood as offering them a role in life, an opportunity to be the centre of attention, and the unconditional love of another human being. Some of these (but not all) will have chaotic lifestyles and be far from able to provide a baby and young child with the secure routines that help them thrive. Just as with older women, some young women get pregnant because they think it will help them keep their boyfriend, or because having a baby confers on them 'womanhood' and raises them in their own esteem and others'. Some teenagers will be shocked by their pregnancy, but use it to plan for a future for themselves and their baby that will ensure the wellbeing of both. They will be motivated by early parenthood to gain qualifications, find a first or better job, and identify and make use of new opportunities available to them as mothers.

Whatever the educator thinks are the reasons behind the pregnancies of the young mothers attending her/his programme, they will probably not be the only reasons, or not the reasons at all.

The state of mind of a pregnant teenager is likely to be complex with fear rubbing shoulders with anxiety, confusion, loneliness and frustration as well as excitement and joy. The young mother's neurobiological development is far from complete and important facets of behaviour such as impulse control, self-regulation and the ability not to give in to the desire for instant gratification, as well as being able to plan and anticipate the consequences of actions, are still emerging (Steinberg et al., 2009; Giedd et al., 2015).

While the pregnancy may be a young woman's way of rebelling or challenging assumptions about herself or a creative search for change and meaning, it will also bring with it fears about life and death, and a growing realisation that the boundaries she had hoped to leap over by virtue of being pregnant will be replaced by other boundaries that cannot be circumvented. Restrictions on what she can eat or drink during pregnancy may be ignored (but doing so will bring feelings of guilt and worry) or adhered to, but regretfully so as peers continue to drink and party. Parents from whom the young person wanted to escape may suddenly have to assume a much bigger part in her life because of the need for financial support, perhaps a roof over her head, and babysitting services.

All of the above may explain why young mothers are at significantly higher risk of depression and anxiety disorders than older ones (McCracken & Loveless, 2014), with self-harm being a common feature of their profile. It has been estimated that more than half of young mothers suffer from perinatal mental health problems (Reid & Meadows-Oliver, 2007).

Young mothers are at risk of depression and anxiety disorders, with self-harm being common. It has been estimated that more than half of young mothers suffer from perinatal mental health problems.

Into practice

This chapter considers birth and parenting education for young mothers who are not in need of the more intensive support and education provided by programmes such as the Family Nurse Partnership (called the Nurse Family Partnership in the USA). However, it may become apparent to educators while running 'standard' groups for young mothers that some need far more support than the group can offer and should be referred.

Aims of early parenting education for young mothers

It is important to be clear about the aims of parenting education sessions for young mothers. Formulating these aims, agreeing them with all colleagues who will be involved in the programme and keeping them constantly in mind during each session and when reflecting afterwards is a key means of ensuring that sessions are tailored to the specific needs of the young mothers who are attending them.

YoungMumsAid, a South-East London-based service, defines its aims as:

- *To improve the mental health of young mums by increasing their self-confidence, aspirations and sense of agency*
- *To promote better chances of optimal development of babies by improving the quality of bonding and attunement*
- *To reduce social isolation and strengthen support networks.*

(based on Donaghy et al. 2017:17)

There are some clear 'no-no's' when it comes to leading groups for young clients. Criticism is never taken well; even the smallest hint of it may result in an outburst, or secret resentment, with the mother leaving the group and perhaps not returning. So, educators must constantly censor the words that are coming out of their mouth in order to ensure respect for the mothers' sometimes hair-trigger sensitivities. The educator is aiming to help them express their ideas about becoming a new mum, ideas that are probably in the making rather than fully formed, which may be difficult to formulate, and a constant revelation to the young woman herself as they take shape. The group presents the opportunity, if facilitated with patience and a strong ability to listen, for young mothers to understand themselves better by sharing thoughts and feelings with their peers and reflecting on and empathising with other people's ideas. Young mothers are well supported when the educator honestly acknowledges the difficulties of pregnancy and early parenthood and helps them to form reasonable expectations of babies and mothering. She therefore needs to avoid offering her own 'solutions' to the difficulties the young women face, and instead, help them to find their own way forward.

Defining group membership

Who exactly are 'young mothers' needs defining in the context of early parenting education because approaches to teaching and learning that are suitable for thirteen- and fourteen-year-olds may be very different from those appropriate for eighteen- or nineteen-year-olds. The educator's aim of building a peer support network may be thwarted if young people at very different stages of their physical, social and emotional development are grouped together. The phrase 'teenage pregnancy' excludes young mothers in their early twenties, yet these women may still be vulnerable in many of the same respects as their younger peers, that is, financially insecure, unsupported, lacking in qualifications, still in the process of becoming autonomous, self-determining adults. Educators need to be clear with colleagues who may recruit young mothers into their early education programmes about the age range their programme is intended for.

> It is important to be clear about the age range for which the early parenting programme is intended as the needs and circumstances of young teenagers are different from those of older ones, and thirteen-year-olds do not mix socially with eighteen-year-olds.

Continuity of educator

Early parenting education offers young mothers the opportunity to form a relationship with an educator who can be a 'still point of the turning world' as they negotiate the transition to parenthood. Continuity of educator is more important for this group than for general parent education groups. Meeting the same educator each week from mid-pregnancy through to the first months of their baby's life can provide a basis of security for young women that may have been entirely lacking in their lives to date, and the reassurance that they are not being abandoned to cope on their own.

> The same educator facilitating every session in the early parenting programme can provide a secure base for young women making the transition to parenthood.

Challenging and being challenged

Early parenting education can bring out the best and the worst – both in the young people who attend the sessions and in those who lead them.

Adolescence is a period when it is (almost) acceptable and expected to challenge older people, to have one's own ideas, to behave recklessly and to see the world as owing you a good time. Teenagers are still very much in the process of sorting out their relationship with 'authority'. Whether or not the educator presents her- or himself as an authority figure, s/he will be perceived and labelled by young parents, at least initially, as such. Depending on their personality, experiences and the stage they are at in the process of growing up, young mothers may kick against any and every piece of advice they are offered by older people, or may accept it word for word and implement it in a literal manner that allows for no modification according to circumstances. Some young mothers who appear to be highly dismissive of what is being discussed may, in fact, be storing information away diligently and act on some or much of it later on. Teenagers may show extraordinary insight into their situation or appear to be wilfully or helplessly oblivious to what is happening to them. Some will be disruptive in the group, although this is certainly less common than educators fear as participants have often had to find a great deal of courage to come to the group in the first place and are highly motivated to learn about their babies.

Educators may be challenged by young mothers' groups in ways that they find hard to explain. Unacknowledged grief around the loss of their own youth may be expressed either in a punitive attitude towards their young clients, or in an unhelpfully liberal approach to their current pregnancies and imminent parenthood. The young mothers' sometimes risky lifestyles may grate on educators' mature sense of appropriate behaviour. There may be other difficult feelings for educators – in some circumstances, anger that these young people are having babies so 'easily' when perhaps they themselves or their close friends have had difficulty in conceiving; irritation at the young mothers' perceived irresponsibility; frustration about their apparent lack of understanding of the huge responsibilities they are undertaking; and despair that they are about to take charge of a helpless, vulnerable human being.

It is, of course, important to put all these feelings to one side and to be with the young parents in an accepting, non-judgemental and mindful way. Young mothers need educators to demonstrate:

- *Reliability and trustworthiness*
- *Non-judgemental listening*
- *Empathy without intrusion (neither under-involved nor over-identified)*
- *A realistic understanding of their circumstances*
- *Willingness to engage with fathers-to-be and other family members (as appropriate).*

(based on Otley 2015:20)

Achieving the right level of engagement requires constant reflection and the support of a colleague with whom the educator can talk through her feelings, gain insights into issues that are 'pressing buttons', and to:

- *Acknowledge and contain the emotional impact of working with a cohort of parents and their babies who live with high levels of need and in close proximity to vulnerability*
- *Ensure that child protection and safeguarding of the baby and mother remain a focus in practice* (Andrews & Oxley, 2015:25)
- *Enhance the knowledge and confidence of the educator and her ability to apply learning in practice with the ultimate aim of improving outcomes for the client and her unborn baby.*

It is beyond the remit of this book to explore issues relating to child protection; educators leading groups for young women potentially affected by safeguarding concerns will be supported by protocols drawn up by the institutions for which they work, and, hopefully, mandatory supervisory sessions to provide them with the support they themselves require to be able to support the young mothers.

Active listening

Active listening is important when facilitating groups for young mothers who may find difficulty in expressing themselves or who may express themselves very easily but without much reflection on what they are saying. Educators can reflect their ideas back to them:

- *So, what you are saying is …. Is that right?*
- *Let me make sure I understand what your point is ….*
- *I think you feel that …*
- *So are you agreeing with what (name) said or do you feel differently?*

Rather than challenging misconceptions from a position of authority as leader of the group, it can be helpful to enlist the group itself in countering mistaken information and negative ideas:

- *What have other people in the group heard about 'eating for two' in pregnancy?*
- *Does anyone in the group know of someone who has found breastfeeding easy? What worked for them?*
- *I'd like to hear what other people in the group think about this – it's such an important topic.*

Keeping the baby in mind

The *baby's* point of view needs to be kept in mind at all times. The educator can ask parents what the baby might consider to be an ideal mother, and what the baby would most like from his parents as he grows up. Thinking about how the baby might be experiencing the world both in utero and when he is very young is a central tenet of mentalisation – trying to understand how the baby is making sense of the world in which he is living.

> The educator needs to make sure that the *baby's* point of view is kept in mind throughout the programme.

By taking a strong interest in the young mothers' descriptions of their unborn babies, for example of when the babies are active and when quiet, what they like and dislike in relation to voices and sounds, and their reactions to various foods eaten by their mothers, the educator is acknowledging that all babies are individuals with their own characteristics and preferences. For some of the young mothers, thinking of their babies as distinct from themselves may be novel. The educator helps them to build a relationship with their unborn babies through exploring and delighting in their individuality. Early parenting education can help lay the foundations for a postnatal relationship in which the mother focuses on trying to understand her baby's needs on the basis that the baby is a person quite separate and different from herself, although entirely dependent.

Inviting a new mother to visit the group with her baby can provide a role model for young mothers who have had no positive parenting in their lives. A mother who can demonstrate a responsive relationship with her baby in the way that she holds him and talks to him, and talks *about* him, may be a revelation to members of the group. The facilitator will need to choose the visiting mum with care – someone with good interpersonal skills and a sense of humour, who is non-judgemental, who can talk about labour and birth without exaggeration and who is clearly aware of her baby's unique individuality rather than perceiving her relationship with him as a series of activities initiated by herself.

The visiting baby him- or herself is a wonderful 'teaching aid' and can be the trigger for exploring the mother–baby relationship. The educator might ask:

- *Why do you think the baby likes looking at his mum?*
- *What is the baby learning from his mum?*
- *Why does the baby turn her head away sometimes when she's been looking at her mum?*
- *What do the baby's movements tell her mum about how she's feeling?*

The mother can describe 'typical' days with her baby, thus helping develop reasonable expectations on the part of the young mothers about their postnatal lives, and can discuss how she manages tiredness and avoids isolation.

Relationship education

Relationship education is a key feature of sessions for young mothers. Many young women may have been in abusive relationships, or still are, especially those who come from impoverished backgrounds (Roosa et al., 1997; Garwood et al., 2015). Their concept of a relationship may accommodate violence perpetrated against them so that they view being slapped or burned with cigarettes and treated contemptuously as a normal part of life with their child's father. Discussions about what makes a good mother, and what makes a good father, and ways in which partners can work together to parent their baby may provide the educator with insights into the difficulties individuals are facing, and the opportunity, therefore, to refer them on. The group itself may provide feedback on the acceptability of incidents that members of the group describe, or beliefs about relationships they put forward. Challenges to long-held and unexplored ideas about relationships may be more acceptable when coming from peers, than from the educator.

Mental health

A recent project focusing on the mental health of young mothers, Young Mums Together, aims:

- *To provide practical, emotional and mental health support to young mothers in the community*
- *To encourage young mothers to connect with mental health professionals, as well as a peer support network*
- *To raise awareness of topics related to mental health and referral routes to services*
- *To remove stigma around issues affecting young mothers.*

The report on the project (Mental Health Foundation, 2018) states that topics of interest to group members were as follows:

- *Stress*
- *Confident parenting*
- *Mental health and mental illness (particularly depression)*
- *Stereotypes and stigmas of 'motherhood'*
- *Mood*
- *Positive social relationships*

- *Communicating with your child*
- *Sexual health and safety.*

Early parenting groups for young mothers need to talk about mental health because:

> Young mothers are at a higher risk of postpartum depression than average, which is associated with feelings of isolation and low self-esteem. Postpartum depression, if unchecked, can have long-term consequences for both the mother and her child. In addition, a lack of support with mental health difficulties can have negative effects on parenting practices and can affect the mother's ability to bond with her child.
>
> (Mental Health Foundation 2018)

General discussion around positive mental health, highlighting everyday measures for maintaining a positive outlook, may be preventative for some of the young mothers in the group. Discussion may be initiated by questions such as:

- *What makes you happy in your lives?*
- *What makes you unhappy?*
- *What is the difference between having a bad day and being depressed?*
- *How do you avoid becoming depressed?*
- *If you are depressed, what can you do about it?*
- *Who can help and how can they help?*
- *What support is available for young parents?*
- *What groups can you go to?*
- *Where can you get advice?*
- *Where can you get practical help?*

Discussion in which personal experiences of depression are shared, or those of others in relation to having a baby, may alert the educator to individuals who would benefit from further support.

Doing everything possible to help the young mothers develop a support network from the group is a primary means of promoting positive mental health. This may be harder to achieve than with a group of older, more settled women and couples. Young parents may lack social skills, be suspicious of other young women, have 'history' with each other or simply not trust anyone as they have learned that most people whom they meet are not dependable. It will take time for young mothers to form truly supportive relationships, and become willing and able to offer each other sensitive emotional and practical support. It is not possible to nurture a sense of kinship that will endure beyond the group's life if the educator has only a single session or a couple of sessions with the group. Early parenting programmes for young mothers therefore need to run over many months from pregnancy through to the early weeks of the babies' lives.

The educator should aim to help the young mothers develop a support network from the group as a primary means of promoting positive mental health and reducing isolation.

Developing question-asking skills

Young women who have had to fight constantly to be heard during their lives may be uncertain as to how to conduct a conversation which is assertive rather than aggressive with a childbirth, early years (or other) professional. Role play in which group participants 'try out' the roles of a mother asking for a particular form of care or intervention, and of a health professional caring for her, can help the group identify what kinds of attitude 'work' and what kinds of questions to ask. A mnemonic such as BRAIN may be helpful for mothers in structuring a discussion, with a midwife, for example, at an antenatal clinic, or during labour:

The BRAIN mnemonic

B: What are the <u>benefits</u> of this treatment/intervention for me and my baby?
R: What are the <u>risks</u> of this treatment/intervention?
A: Is there an <u>alternative</u>?
I: (question to self) What does my <u>instinct</u> tell me about this?
N: What would happen if we did <u>nothing</u>?

The group can think about the kind of childbirth experience they want to have and how to convey their wishes to the midwives and doctors looking after them. The impact of certain ways of expressing themselves on their relationship with professionals can be explored, and strategies for being assertive but maintaining a positive, respectful relationship can be identified. Question-asking skills are not just for labour and birth, but will be essential for the mother as she takes on the responsibility of making decisions for her child.

Budgeting

Many young mothers-to-be will be short of money and parenting education provides a great opportunity to help develop budgeting skills. A structured format for thinking about expenditure and income is provided in the appendix at the end of the book ('General family budgeting'). Talking about how to save money will also lead to group members sharing ideas about where the best bargains are to be found for baby equipment and other essential items. The young mothers themselves will usually prove to be the experts on money-saving tips and the educator can sit back and learn from them.

Signposting

Early parenting programmes for young mothers are likely to reveal a great deal of unmet need in relation to the young women's conditions of daily living and the educator needs to know to whom she can refer them for information about employment and training opportunities, benefits, accommodation, and for mental health support and support with relationship problems. A community venue such as a children's centre is therefore ideal for sessions for young parents, providing a 'one-stop shop' where they can get to know people who can help them, and receive ongoing peer support from other parents attending the centre.

Young fathers

This chapter has talked about early parenting groups for young *mothers* because there is a considerable body of research and practice experience to inform understanding of their needs, and of their preferred means of acquiring information and skills in preparation for parenting. Academic interest in young fathers has been far less vigorous. It is only in recent years that fathers in general have become a focus of research and that their needs have been better identified and met, largely owing to the strong advocacy of fathers themselves through organisations such as The Fatherhood Institute in the UK. Attracting young men to sessions may be difficult. Approaching them in settings that are not specifically educational may be the best way of starting a relationship and interesting them in parenting education. For example, talking to young fathers at the antenatal clinic, especially if the approach is made by a male healthcare professional or youth worker, to offer support may be an effective way of informing them about parenting education.

Running dedicated groups for young fathers can require a lot of effort and resilience on the part of the educator:

> *Getting in touch with the young fathers and the initial conversations can be difficult. I have had young men express suspicion as to why a complete stranger would want to offer them support in relation to being a dad ... Sometimes, a dad whom I have tried to engage for several months will turn up to a weekly group unannounced. I have often been told that the reason for this change of heart is the regular texts I send out about the sessions. One young father told me that the reason he was initially hesitant to engage was*

because of the negative reactions he had had from his friends, family and teachers when he had announced the news that he was going to be a dad. He was curious as to why a stranger would call him up and be thrilled for him, and offer him the chance to share his excitement with other expectant and new fathers when no one else in his life had shown any interest in the matter.

(O'Kane 2014:33)

Inviting a father to visit an early parenting group with his baby and talk about his feelings for his child and how he is involved in her care may help young fathers begin to define a role for themselves that they had neither anticipated nor hoped for or perhaps wanted. Where young fathers can be positively engaged with their child, even if the relationship with the mother is short-term, or already over, has been shown to have benefits. In a study (Lewin et al., 2015) of young mothers suffering from depression, 78% of the fathers of their children were engaged with them, typically seeing their baby a few times each month, and 71% took some financial responsibility for their child. Father engagement predicted lower infant distress, and buffered the effect of maternal depression on the baby. The authors concluded that fathers may be a protective resource for children born to teen mothers, potentially mitigating the heightened risks associated with maternal depression in the postpartum period.

Key points

Research and theory

- Babies of teenage mothers are at increased risk of low birthweight, of being stillborn, of dying in infancy, and of not being breastfed
- Young mothers are more likely than older mothers not to be in education, employment or training, to be care-leavers, to have experienced physical and emotional abuse, and to be living in poverty
- It has been estimated that more than half of young mothers suffer from perinatal mental health problems
- Engaged fathers may be a protective resource for children born to teen mothers, potentially mitigating the heightened risks associated with maternal depression in the postpartum period

Into practice

- Educators need to be clear about the age range their programme is intended for
- Continuity of educator is important for young mothers' groups, providing a basis of security for women who may have had little experience of being nurtured

- Educators aim to improve the mental health of young mums by increasing the mothers' self-confidence, aspirations and sense of agency and by developing the group as a support network
- The educator needs to avoid offering her/his own 'solutions' to the difficulties the young mothers face and, instead, help them to find their own way forward
- A visiting mother and baby are a wonderful 'teaching aid' for exploring the mother–baby relationship
- Exploring couple relationships and how partners can work together as parents is a key aspect of early parenting education
- Highlighting everyday measures for maintaining positive mental health may be preventative for some young mothers
- Early parenting education provides an opportunity to help young mothers develop budgeting skills
- The educator needs to know to whom she can refer young mothers for information about employment and training opportunities, benefits, accommodation, and for support with their mental health and with relationship problems

Note

In the Appendix are teaching activities, 'Exploring mental health', 'Myths and realities about babies', 'What do you want for your baby? What does your baby need?' and 'General family budgeting', which may be helpful in facilitating sessions for young mothers.

References

Andrews, L., Oxley, A. (2015/16) Supervision in FNP: A reflection on practice. *International Journal of Birth and Parent Education*, 3(2):25-28.

Donaghy, M., McGuinness, S., Smith, K. (2017) Supporting young mothers. *International Journal of Birth & Parent Education*, 4(3):17-20.

Garwood, S.K., Gerassi, L., Jonson-Reid, M., Plax, K., Drake, B. (2015) More than poverty: The effect of child abuse and neglect on teen pregnancy risk. *Journal of Adolescent Health*, 57(2):164-168.

Giedd, J.N., Raznahan, A., Alexander-Bloch, A., Schmitt, E., Gogtay, N. et al. (2015) Child psychiatry branch of the National Institute of Mental Health longitudinal structural magnetic resonance imaging study of human brain development. *Neuropsychopharmacology*, 40(1):43-49.

Lewin, A., Mitchell, S.J., Waters, D., Hodgkinson, S., Southammakosane, C. et al. (2015) The protective effects of father involvement for infants of teen mothers with depressive symptoms. *Maternal and Child Health Journal*, 19:1016-1023.

McCracken, K.A., Loveless, M. (2014) Teen pregnancy: An update. *Current Opinion in Obstetrics and Gynecology*, 26:355-359.

McDermott, E., Graham, H. (2005) Resilient young mothering: Social inequalities, late modernity and the 'problem' of 'teenage' motherhood. *Journal of Youth Studies*, 8(10):59-79.

Mental Health Foundation (2018) *Young Mums Together: Promoting Young Mothers' Wellbeing*. Available at: www.mentalhealth.org.uk/sites/default/files/young-mums-together-report.pdf (accessed 8 July 2018).

Office for National Statistics (2018) Conceptions in England and Wales: 2016. ONS. Available at: www.ons.gov.uk/peoplepopulationandcommunity/birthsdeathsandmarriages/conceptionandfertilityrates/bulletins/conceptionstatistics/2016 (accessed 4 July 2018).

O'Kane, S. (2014) Engaging young fathers. *International Journal of Birth and Parent Education*, 1(3):33-34.

Otley, H. (2015) A psychodynamic approach to working with pregnant teenagers and young parents. *International Journal of Birth and Parent Education*, 2(4):19-21.

Public Health England (2016) *A Framework for Supporting Teenage Mothers and Young Fathers*. London: Public Health England.

Reid, V., Meadows-Oliver, M. (2007) Postpartum depression in adolescent mothers: An integrative review of the literature. *Journal of Paediatric Health Care*, 21:289-298.

Roosa, M.W., Tein, J-Y., Reinholtz, C., Angelini, P.J. (1997) The relationship of childhood sexual abuse to teenage pregnancy. *Journal of Marriage and Family*, 59(1):119-130.

Steinberg, L., Graham, S., O'Brien, L., Woolard, J., Cauffman, E. et al. (2009) Age differences in future orientation and delay discounting. *Child Development*, 80(1):28-44.

Swann, C., Bowe, K., McCormick, G., Kosmin, M. (2003) *Teenage Pregnancy and Parenthood: Evidence Briefing*. London: Health Development Agency.

16 Education and support for mothers and fathers in prison

Imagine anticipating the birth of your child. You have two weeks until the due date, yet the excitement you should feel is overshadowed by anxiety and stress. You are in prison, coping with a restricted diet, limited information and the knowledge that your baby may be taken away from you immediately after birth. This is the reality for some women who find themselves pregnant and in prison.

(Abbott 2016a)

Research and theory

Women make up around 5% of the overall prison population in the UK. The number of women in prison in England and Wales stood at 4035 on 17 November 2017 (Women in Prison, 2017). There are twelve women's prisons in England, none in Wales and one in Scotland. Six prisons have Mother and Baby Units (Prison Life, undated). On average, there will be 600 pregnant women prisoners at any given time, and around two babies a week will be born while their mothers are serving a prison sentence (NSPCC & Barnardo's, 2014).

Unlike many other countries, the UK does not make sentencing allowances for pregnant women in the criminal justice system. Following the birth, some are allowed to keep their baby with them in a prison Mother and Baby Unit until the infant is eighteen months old. Others have their baby taken from them shortly after birth and he or she is placed either with a family member or becomes a looked-after child who may be fostered or adopted. Women are generally held in standard prison cells while pregnant. They are escorted to antenatal appointments and scans by prison guards and transferred to local maternity units for labour and birth, before returning to prison or to a Mother and Baby Unit (Fenton, 2016).

On average, there are 600 pregnant women in prison at any given time in England and Wales, and around two babies a week are born while their mothers are serving a prison sentence.

It is surprising and concerning that, in an era of abundant, easy-to-access information, there are no figures for the number of fathers in prison. However, over half (54%) of the 1435 male prisoners interviewed for a Ministry of Justice study published in 2012 had children under the age of eighteen at the time they entered prison (cited in Prison Reform Trust, 2013). There are also no exact statistics available for the number of babies and toddlers in prison in the UK. Nor are there any precise figures for the number of children whose mother or father is in prison, or how old they are. The Prison Reform Trust estimates that approximately 200,000 children in England and Wales had a parent in prison at some point in 2009 (latest figure available). This is more than double the number of children affected in the same year by divorce (Prison Reform Trust, 2013). The courts, government and local social services do not routinely ask about the children of convicted women and men and so they often remain hidden from services. Yet children of prisoners are twice as likely as children without an incarcerated parent to experience conduct and mental health problems, and less likely to do well at school (Barnardo's, 2019).

Prisoners, whether male or female, are a highly vulnerable population. They are likely to have experienced trauma in childhood, ranging from physical, emotional and sexual abuse to poverty and frequent change of caregiver, and to have been alcohol- and/or drug-dependent since adolescence. In a Scottish study (Karatzias et al., 2018) of eighty-nine female prisoners, 91% of the women reported both child and adult trauma. An Australian study (Martin et al., 2015) of 5154 male prisoners found that 45% of inmates reported childhood trauma, and amongst these, there was a higher prevalence of mental health and substance abuse needs, and youth criminal charges, than in the rest of the prison population. A third of people assessed in prison in 2017–2018 reported that they had a learning disability or difficulty (Prison Reform Trust: Bromley Briefings, 2019).

Mental health problems are rife in the prison population. Recent figures from the Prison Reform Trust (2013) reveal that 26% of women and 16% of men have received treatment for a mental health problem in the year before custody, and a quarter of female and 15% of male prisoners report symptoms of psychosis. Suicide is nearly nine times more likely amongst prisoners than in the general population.

Mental health problems are highly prevalent in the prison population.

Women who are pregnant in prison are undergoing the physical and emotional challenges of pregnancy in an often hostile environment and far away from friends and family. Imprisoned fathers-to-be may be worried about how their pregnant partner is managing on the outside and whether she is able to access the care and afford the items that she needs for the baby. Pregnant women may be especially fearful that their baby will not be able to stay with them while they serve out the rest of their term. In the UK, only about half of women who give birth in prison are able to have a place on a Mother and Baby Unit (Abbott, 2016b). Even in a Mother and Baby Unit, staff may not be especially knowledgeable about babycare.

Parenting a new baby in prison is clearly very difficult, given the lack of privacy, strict and inflexible routines, lack of choice of food, lack of access to professional advice and lack of support from key people in the woman's outside world. Imprisoned fathers who have a new baby at home may feel guilty about not being able to provide support and distressed that they are not present to share their baby's first days, weeks and months, and all the changes that happen in the first year of life.

Whether babies are with their mothers in prison, have a father in prison or have been removed from their mothers and placed with foster families, they inevitably:

> encounter risks that could affect their care and development. This occurs for a number of reasons. Firstly, those involved in the criminal justice system often have additional needs, such as poor mental health, that can impact on the care the baby receives. Secondly, the criminal justice system can disrupt relationships, particularly if parents and infants are separated. Thirdly, the physical incarceration of pregnant women and babies in Mother and Baby Units can impact on the health and wellbeing of infants.
>
> (NSPCC & Barnardo's 2014:5)

Into practice

The 2014 report from the NSPCC in conjunction with Barnardo's, *An Unfair Sentence: All Babies Count: Spotlight on the Criminal Justice System*, made several recommendations in relation to parenting education:

- *Parenting programmes delivered in prisons should be evidence based, delivered by trained specialist staff and available to all. Parenting programmes should include face to face support as well as online programmes, address parental needs and promote sensitive caregiving.*
- *There should be parenting support programmes available to all fathers in prison to support bonding and to promote attachment relationships between fathers in prison and their new babies, as well as to support their relationship*

with their partners (where appropriate). These should be adapted as appropriate for different target groups, for example for young men.

- In prisons, parenting education and activities should be formally recognised as part of 'prison-based activities' (Scotland) and 'sentence-planning activities' (England and Wales) in recognition that they may reduce the risk of reoffending and support resettlement.
- There should be a continuous focus on learning and improving the quality of the provision of parenting programmes for parents and babies through rigorous evaluation. (p39)

The Albertson review (2012) noted that minimal antenatal education was one of the deficits experienced by pregnant women prisoners. Karatzias et al. (2018:abstract) recommended that, 'When women or girls are sent to prison, the opportunity for constructive interventions must be seized'. The provision of early parenting education in a prison requires careful preparation and negotiation with the prison authorities. Educators need to make preliminary visits to the prison to talk to staff and find out the profile of prisoners who are pregnant or parents, what services are available to them, for example to help them manage alcohol or substance abuse problems, and how staff feel about parenting education. If educators show themselves eager to understand how the prison operates and what their role in it might be, staff are more likely to take an interest in the work they want to do and may express an interest in observing sessions. Key personnel with whom UK educators should try to establish a positive relationship are the Family Engagement Worker and local representatives of the Prison Advice and Care Trust (PACT). Educators should also consult materials used in recognised interventions, such as Fathers Inside, an intensive group work programme for men and young men in prison which focuses on parental responsibilities and children's development and wellbeing. Programmes that aim to improve the environment of relationships into which the baby will be born should include both the incarcerated parent and the 'outside' parent, whenever possible.

Prison-based early parenting education programmes aim to:

- Improve the quality of interaction between mothers/fathers and their babies
- Increase mothers'/fathers' confidence in their ability to parent their babies
- Decrease levels of anxiety and stress around parenting
- Foster a positive, respectful, co-parenting partnership between the incarcerated parent and the 'outside' parent (where it is possible for couples to attend sessions together in the prison).

Content may include:

- Practical babycare skills such as feeding, soothing, bathing, changing nappies
- Baby massage
- Understanding babies' behaviour and development

- *Talking to babies, singing and reading*
- *What it means to be a mother/father*
- *Managing the stress of parenting*
- *Signposts to organisations and centres offering support following discharge.*

The need for educators to be flexible is paramount. Group sessions will have to accommodate women who are at various stages of pregnancy, as well as women who have just given birth or who gave birth some months previously. This is because it is unlikely that there will be sufficient pregnant women and new mothers to run groups more specifically tailored to a particular stage of the transition to parenthood. However, this diversity in terms of the stage at which each prisoner is on her journey to parenthood offers opportunity for more experienced parents to share ideas with and support those who are pregnant for the first time or who have a new baby.

Groups for male prisoners are likely to be similarly diverse, including men who are awaiting the birth of their child, men who have a new baby at home and men who are father to one or more young children.

Educators also need to be prepared for groups to be a fluctuating population as participants finish their sentences or are transferred to other prisons, or are unable to attend because they have to perform duties in the prison or attend other meetings. Each session therefore needs to be self-contained with learning outcomes clearly identified so that the educator can feel confident that s/he has supported every participant to acquire knowledge and skills that will be valuable should they not be able to join the group again.

Early parenting groups in prison are likely to include women and men who have learning difficulties. Educators need therefore to be prepared to cut back their usual programmes and to identify and focus on key learning outcomes. Hands-on activities with dolls such as practising bathing, changing and soothing can incorporate discussion of interacting with babies and how to meet babies' emotional as well as their physical needs.

Informed choices: labour and birth

While any early parenting programme aims to support women to make their own choices about how they want to give birth to their baby, whether they want to go to the maternity unit as early as possible in labour or as late, who they would like to be with them, and how they would like to spend the first hours of their baby's life, many of these 'informed choices' are simply not available to mothers who, for example, can only go to hospital in labour when arrangements have been made to take them there in secure transport. Nor can women prisoners make choices about the kind of maternity unit (obstetric-led, alongside or freestanding midwife-led unit) in which they would like to give birth, or the things they would like to take with them, such as pillows, bean bags or birthing balls. For women prisoners, breastfeeding may also not be a choice if their baby is likely to be removed from them soon after birth.

It's important, therefore, to build a sense of agency by emphasising the choices that do lie within the women's remit. They can be helped to make a choice, for example, about what kind of pain relief they would like in labour. If their choice is to labour without pain-relieving drugs, educators need to help them understand how to manage contractions using breathing techniques, affirmations and remaining upright and mobile. Like all other mothers, women prisoners can ask to have protected skin-to-skin time with their new baby. It is their right to make requests and ask questions about the care they want or are receiving, although some women will need help to understand how to question assertively rather than aggressively. Role play as described in Chapter 15 (see section: Developing question-asking skills) may be useful to explore the impact of different ways of asking questions.

> Educators can build a sense of agency by emphasising the childbirth choices that women prisoners *can* make.

Supporting mental health

The prevalence of all mental disorders is higher in prisoners than in the general population (Fazel et al., 2016) and the children of parents who suffer from mental health problems are at increased risk of developing mental ill health themselves (Mental Health Foundation, 2016). Early parenting education in prison provides an opportunity to transmit mental health messages, although as educators get to know their clients better, they may become very aware that some need far more mental health care than it is possible to provide in their sessions. Nonetheless, basic messages about maintaining positive mental health can be discussed. The Mental Health Foundation (online) makes the following suggestions, although some of these are not under the control of prisoners and will be relevant only following release:

- *Find someone you can talk to about your feelings*
- *Keep active because activity increases your endorphins (happy hormones)*
- *Eat a diet that contains some fruit and vegetables*
- *Use alcohol in moderation*
- *Keep in touch with friends*
- *Take a break – even if just for five minutes – from doing things you find difficult or boring*

- *Make time to do things you're good at, such as painting, or making things with the children, or cooking a meal*
- *Help other people*
- *Accept who you are. Like everyone else, there are good things about you and things that you wish you could change. Everyone is the same*
- *Ask for help if you are feeling very low and just can't cope.*

(Mental Health Foundation online)

Many mothers are in prison for only a short term; it's therefore vital to include in every session information about where they can go for support following discharge. A list of organisations offering help to ex-prisoners and their families can be handed out to all new participants at the first session as they may only be able to come to a single session:

UK organisations which support prisoners and their families

- *Action for Prisoners' and Offenders' Families: Supports families who are affected by imprisonment*
- *Birth Companions: Aims to make pregnancy, birth and motherhood a positive experience for women prisoners*
- *PACT (Prison Advice and Care Trust): Provides support to prisoners, people with convictions and their families to make a fresh start, and minimise the harm that can be caused by imprisonment*
- *POPS (Partners of Prisoners): Established by offenders' families for offenders' families – identifies needs and finds the solutions*

The educator has to take responsibility for ensuring that the list is regularly updated and, if possible, should provide contact details for resources in the particular areas from which group participants come. It is obviously important to avoid a newly discharged and possibly desperate mother ringing a number that is no longer in use, or contacting a support group that folded some months previously.

Conclusion

The challenges of providing early parenting education in prison are considerable; the opportunities are rewarding. The educator aims 'to capitalize on the unique opportunity for positive life change that is offered by the prospect of becoming a mother' (Shaw et al., 2015:1460) or a father. Men and women prisoners are usually eager to ensure that their children have a better start in life than they themselves had and receive better parenting. They are therefore highly motivated to understand how to relate to their babies and toddlers so that their children can enjoy a different and more joyful relationship with them than they had with their own parents. The educator can make a positive contribution to participants' self-esteem by the way in which s/he respects their status as a mother or father. This is key as, 'parents in prison report feeling defined more by their prisoner status than by their impending parenthood owing to the lack of acknowledgement of pregnancy in prison' (Coster & Brookes, 2017:15). The early parenting group provides a space where imprisoned mothers and fathers may be able to relax and feel that their parenthood is valued.

Key points

Research and theory

- On average in England and Wales, there are 600 pregnant women prisoners at any given time, and around two babies a week are born while their mothers are serving a sentence. There are no figures for the number of fathers in prison
- Prisoners are a highly vulnerable population. They are likely to have experienced trauma in childhood, ranging from physical, emotional and sexual abuse, to poverty and frequent change of caregiver, and to have been alcohol- and/or drug-dependent since adolescence
- The prevalence of all mental disorders is higher in prisoners than in the general population
- The incarceration of pregnant women and babies in Mother and Baby Units can impact on the health and wellbeing of infants
- Parenting a new baby in prison is very difficult owing to lack of privacy, strict and inflexible routines, lack of choice of food, lack of access to professional advice and lack of support from the woman's family

Into practice

- Educators intending to offer early parenting education in prison need to make preliminary visits to talk to staff and find out the profile of prisoners who are pregnant or parents, what services are available to them and how staff feel about parenting education
- Early parenting education programmes that aim to improve the environment of relationships into which the baby will be born should ideally include both the incarcerated parent and the 'outside' parent, whenever possible

- Group sessions need to accommodate women who are at various stages of pregnancy, as well as women who have recently given birth, as it is unlikely that there will be sufficient pregnant women and new mothers to run groups specifically tailored to a particular stage of the transition to parenthood
- Educators need to be prepared for groups to be a fluctuating population as participants finish their sentences or are transferred to other prisons, or are unable to attend because they have duties in the prison or other meetings
- It is important to build women's sense of agency by identifying birth choices that lie within their remit
- Early parenting education in prison provides an excellent opportunity to transmit mental health messages
- Many mothers are in prison for only a short term; therefore every session needs to include information about where women can go for support following discharge

Note

In the Appendix are teaching activities, 'Exploring mental health', 'Myths and realities about babies', 'What do you want for your baby? What does your baby need?' and 'General family budgeting', which may be helpful in facilitating sessions for mothers in prison.

References

Abbott, L. (2016a) Prison is a stressful place for pregnant women, but with help the service can improve. *The Conversation*. Available at: https://theconversation.com/prison-is-a-stressful-place-for-pregnant-women-but-with-help-the-service-can-improve-58465 (accessed 21 October 2019).

Abbott, L. (2016b) Becoming a mother in prison. *The Practising Midwife*, 19(9):1-3.

Albertson, K., O'Keefe, C., Lessing-Turner, G., Burke, C., Renfrew, M. (2012) *Tackling Health Inequalities Through Developing Evidence-Based Policy and Practice with Childbearing Women in Prison: A Consultation*. Sheffield: The Hallam Centre for Community Justice: Sheffield Hallam University and the Mother and Infant Research Unit at the University of York.

Barnardo's (2019) *Children with a Parent in Prison*. Available at: www.barnardos.org.uk/what_we_do/our_work/children_of_prisoners.htm (accessed 22 July 2019).

Coster, D., Brookes, H. (2017) Perinatal education needs of imprisoned mothers and fathers. *International Journal of Birth and Parent Education*, 4(3):14-16.

Fazel, S., Hayes, A.J., Bartellas, K., Clerici, M., Trestman, R. (2016) Mental health of prisoners: Prevalence, adverse outcomes and interventions. *The Lancet Psychiatry*, 3(9):871-881.

Fenton, S. (2016) The women forced to give birth in front of prison guards. Available at:www.independent.co.uk/news/uk/crime/prison-pregnant-women-babies-significant-harm-public-safety-a7049301.html (accessed 2 July 2018).

Karatzias, T., Power, K., Woolston, C., Apurva, P., Begley, A. et al. (2018) Multiple traumatic experiences, post-traumatic stress disorder and offending behaviour in female prisoners. *Child & Family Social Work*, 28(1):72–84.

Martin, M.S., Eljdupovic, G., McKenzie, K., Colman, I. (2015) Risk of violence by inmates with childhood trauma and mental health needs. *Law and Human Behavior*, 39(6):614–623.

Mental Health Foundation (2016) *Fundamental Facts about Mental Health 2016*. Available at:www.mentalhealth.org.uk/sites/default/files/fundamental-facts-about-mental-health-2016.pdf (accessed 4 July 2018).

Mental Health Foundation (undated) *How to Look After Your Mental Health*. Available at: www.mentalhealth.org.uk/publications/how-to-mental-health (accessed 3 July 2018).

NSPCC & Barnardo's (2014) *An Unfair Sentence. All Babies Count: Spotlight on the Criminal Justice System*. Available at: www.barnardos.org.uk/an-unfair-sentence.pdf (accessed 2 March 2019).

Prison Life (undated) Available at: www.gov.uk/life-in-prison/pregnancy-and-childcare-in-prison (accessed 15 July 2018).

Prison Reform Trust: Bromley Briefings (2019) *Prison: The Facts*. Available at: www.prisonreformtrust.org.uk/portals/0/documents/prisonthefacts.pdf (accessed 22 July 2019).

Prison Reform Trust (2013) *Mental Health Care in Prisons*. Available at:www.prisonreformtrust.org.uk/WhatWeDo/Projectsresearch/Mentalhealth (accessed 22 July 2019).

Shaw, J., Downe, S., Kingdon, C. (2015) Systematic mixed-methods review of interventions, outcomes and experiences for imprisoned pregnant women. *Journal of Advanced Nursing*, 71(7):1451–1463.

Women in Prison (2017) *Key Facts*. Available at: www.womeninprison.org.uk/research/key-facts.php (accessed 2 July 2018).

17 Education and support for at-home parents in military families

Military families in which either one or both parents are serving in the armed forces encounter several obstacles to providing a secure milieu for their young children, challenges that are not usually experienced by civilian families. As a consequence, the children's development may be negatively affected during these critical years.

(Nolan & Misca 2018:10)

Research and theory

Women and men who are serving in the armed forces, or who are the partner of someone who is serving, face particular challenges in their day-to-day lives as parents. The cycle of deployment (pre-deployment, deployment, post-deployment) makes considerable demands on parental resources and challenges the adjustment and wellbeing of children (Creech et al., 2014) (Table 17.1). In the pre-deployment phase, the serving and the at-home parent are preparing emotionally and practically for a potentially long separation. If their child or children are old enough to understand, they, too, must be prepared in an age-appropriate way for the fact that they will not be seeing their father or mother for a while.

During the deployment phase, the at-home parent, usually the mother, becomes, in effect, a single parent, running the household on her own, and caring for the child/ren. In addition, she must cope with constant anxiety about the safety and wellbeing of her partner. Research has shown that at-home parents report elevated levels of emotional distress and problems managing day-to-day activities and relationships (Lara-Cinisomo et al., 2012).

> The military cycle of deployment (pre-deployment, deployment, post-deployment) makes considerable demands on parental resources and challenges the adjustment and wellbeing of children.

The serving parent aims to keep in touch with his or her family, perhaps by email or Skype, but this is not always possible. Apart from the demands of combat, they may worry about how the at-home parent is getting on, and whether the child/ren is/are missing them. Young children may react to the 'loss' of a parent by becoming clingy and reverting to behaviours that they had outgrown, such as needing to sleep with a parent or crying when taken to the child-minder.

In the post-deployment phase, families may experience initial euphoria that the serving parent has returned safely, and that they are indeed a family again; yet, reintegrating the serving parent into a family unit that has functioned well without him or her for several months may be difficult. If the serving parent has returned wounded, physically or psychologically, his or her readjustment will be far more difficult.

In addition to the challenges of the different phases of the cycle of deployment, military families also face regular relocations with the loss of support groups and the need to settle into a different community where they may know nobody.

There is no doubt that some children cope well with military life and enjoy its variety. They may develop skills of self-management and resilience that are not matched by their 'civilian' peers. Nonetheless, research shows that children of military families are at increased risk of social and emotional disturbance (Office for Standards in Educations (Ofsted), 2011). Very young children may become confused, disorientated and demanding as a result of the repeated loss of home environments to which they have become used, and repeated separation from a key caregiver, leaving them highly dependent for their emotional security on the at-home parent who may her- or himself be emotionally fragile (Palmer, 2008). Childen's attachment relationship may be threatened owing to the regular discontinuities in their lives (Schaetti, 2002).

The health and wellbeing of very young children are strongly dependent on the mental health of their primary carers. Research (Mansfield et al., 2010; MacDonell et al., 2016) has shown that at-home parents of military spouses are at increased risk of depression, anxiety, sleep difficulties and psychological disturbances.

Both the at-home parent and the serving parent need support; however, a culture of proud independence and mistrust of sharing emotions persists even today inside the military. The at-home parent may fear seeking help in case this rebounds on her serving partner who is labelled as having a family that cannot cope without him. It is 'a belief widely held by military families that identifying or confirming difficulties can adversely affect the career advancement of the serving parent. This can then lead to reluctance to seek support when difficulties occur' (Lake & Rosan, 2017:27).

Table 17.1 The phases of the deployment cycle: emotional labour of the at-home parent

Deployment cycle	Challenges for at-home parents	Emotional labour
Pre-deployment	Looking ahead Saying goodbye	Planning for the family's future and stability in light of the serving parent's deployment Worrying about how to manage without the serving parent Worrying about the serving parent's safety Facing the departure of the serving member and helping children say goodbye
Deployment	Initial adjustment Parenting from the home front Surviving the home stretch	Adjusting to the absence of the deployed parent Developing routines to manage the home and support children through the separation Looking ahead with a sense of excitement, worry, hope and expectation once the service member's return date is set
Post-deployment	Facing reality Breaking new ground	Creating new or renewed ways of parenting now that the serving parent is home Grappling with new realities when a serving parent is challenged by wartime stressors or injuries Parents continuing to invest in their children through their relationships and parenting efforts as they incorporate deployment-related experiences

(based on Kritikos & DeVoe, 2018:8)

Into practice

Educators working with at-home parents who are pregnant or have very young children and are new to the military may consider inviting experienced parents to join the group who have a lived knowledge and understanding of 'what works' when looking after a 'military family'.

The educator may open a discussion by asking what things give us a sense of security when our lives are disrupted. Participants may suggest that maintaining routines is helpful as an anchor, keeping in touch with loved ones and having a strong support network.

Routines

Young children thrive on routines, and it is likely that children whose lives are often disrupted by the departure of a parent or a move to a new house, a new area or a new country will benefit from having a routine that structures their days. Mindell et al. (2015) note that bedtime routines are especially important in providing security. Children whose parents adhere to a night-time routine that unfolds at the same time and in the same way every night are more settled during the daytime and better able to concentrate. In the military context, Osofsky and Chartrand (2013:68) recommend that at-home parents should 'keep routines consistent and predictable'. The educator can ask the group to suggest a bedtime routine that would be suitable for a six-month baby, a one-year-old and a toddler.

Young children in military families need consistent and predictable routines. A bedtime routine is especially important in promoting security.

Special objects may also provide continuity for young children whatever is happening in their lives. The educator or group members can explain the importance of having much-loved items, such as teddy bears or a comfort blanket, available at bedtime and whenever a move to a new location is made. Pets may also be a very significant part of a young child's life and a source of affection that is constantly available even when the at-home parent is busy or distracted. The educator can emphasise that possessions and pets offer a sense of belonging and stability and are an anchor for identity.

Keeping the serving parent in mind

Very young children have short memories and the at-home parent will want her child to keep the serving parent in mind while the serving parent is on deployment. The educator may initiate a discussion on how this can be achieved. Suggestions may include:

- Showing pictures of the serving parent to the child, especially pictures of the child in the company of or being held by the absent parent
- Playing a recording made prior to the serving parent's deployment of him/ her talking to the child
- Including a story in the bedtime routine that has been recorded by the serving parent prior to deployment
- Telling stories about the serving parent, imagining what s/he is doing and how the family will celebrate when s/he returns. A favourite story may

emerge, developed by the at-home parent and the child, which the child will ask for again and again

- Referring to the serving parent regularly throughout the day.

The educator can explain that stories recorded by the serving parent and stories told by the at-home parent about him/her are very comforting to young children and keep the absent parent 'present' as a positive, playful figure.

Bridges of connection can be built by making drawings, creating a family movie, taking photos of happy moments, and recording stories and songs that can be used at night-time or when the child is particularly sad to bring the deployed parent closer.

(Lieberman & Van Horn 2013:289)

Parents may suggest Skyping as a means of keeping in touch with the deployed parent. Educators should ask whether the group considers that there might be any disadvantages to Skyping, either for themselves or their children. Experienced parents may point out that children could be disturbed by what they see in the background as their parent is talking to them, or they may be frightened if the picture is lost, wondering where the parent 'has gone'. It has been reported by Lincoln and Sweeten (2011) that young children may resort to fantasy when communication is interrupted, and build frightening stories to fill 'the void of limited information'.

Being available to the child

At-home parents can be invited to discuss what kind of behaviour on their part will add to their young children's sense of security. The group will readily acknowledge that their children need them to be available to them, ready to talk and listen, to hold and cuddle them when they're distressed, and play with them. Someone may point out that these are all things that every baby and small child needs, but children in military families may need such contact to be more intense and repeated. The educator can give permission to parents not only to acknowledge their children's sadness at the absence of the serving parent, but also to share their own feelings with their child: 'Mommy is sad because Daddy is gone' (Nolan & Misca, 2018:12). As children develop language, they need to have their emotions named for them, and to start to recognise that others also have emotions that can be named. Openness validates emotions and starts to show young children that it is acceptable and desirable to share their feelings so that they can gain support from key people in their lives.

> The educator can give permission to parents not only to acknowledge their children's sadness at the absence of the serving parent, but also to share their own feelings with their child.

Mental health of the at-home parent

Early parenting education for at-home parents needs to include the opportunity for the group to think carefully about how they can look after themselves through all the phases of the deployment cycle, and where they can find
support. While the military provide many resources for at-home parents, it has
been reported that parents are often unaware of them (Lincoln & Sweeten, 2011).
A group that includes experienced parents alongside first-time parents may be
able to share where and how at-home parents can find help, and the educator
needs to have up-to-date information available to share as s/he would expect to
do with any civilian group. Waliski et al. (2012) advise that peer-to-peer outreach
programmes may be a key strategy for supporting at-home parents with very
young children.

As well as discussing how to access support, the educator will want to invite
parents to think about other ways of maintaining positive mental health; various
approaches have been discussed in other chapters in this book (see especially
Chapters 14, 15 and 16). Experienced parents in the group will be able to tell parents
new to military life about opportunities for socialising, and the times, dates and
venues of parent-and-child groups. Early parenting sessions can themselves provide opportunities for relaxation, helping parents to develop an understanding of
how stress impacts their bodies as well as their minds, and to practise skills for
releasing tension which they can take into their day-to-day lives.

Key points

Research and theory

- The cycle of deployment (pre-deployment, deployment, post-
  deployment) makes considerable demands on parental resources and
  challenges the adjustment and wellbeing of children
- Military families face regular relocations with the loss of support
  groups and the need to settle into different communities where they
  may know nobody
- The child's attachment relationship may be threatened owing to the
  regular discontinuities in her or his life
- At-home parents may be reluctant to seek help in case this rebounds
  on their serving partner

Into practice

- Early parenting education needs to help at-home parents think about
  how they can look after themselves through all the phases of the cycle
  of deployment, and where they can find support

- The educator can draw on the lived understanding of experienced parents in the group who can share 'what works' when looking after a military family
- A discussion can be initiated about the importance of routines for maintaining a sense of security in very young children, and of the significance of special possessions and pets as anchors for identity
- The educator can explain that stories recorded by the serving parent and regularly played while s/he is away keep the absent parent 'present' as a positive figure in their lives
- The educator can give permission to parents to acknowledge their children's sadness at the absence of the serving parent, and also to share their own feelings
- Relaxation education helps parents develop an understanding of how stress impacts their bodies as well as their minds, and includes practising skills for releasing tension which they can take into their day-to-day lives

Note

In the Appendix are teaching activities, 'Exploring mental health', 'Myths and realities about babies' and 'General family budgeting', which may be helpful in facilitating sessions for at-home parents in military families.

References

Creech, S.K., Hadley, W., Borsari, B. (2014) The impact of military deployment and reintegration on children and parenting: A systematic review. *Professional Psychology: Research and Practice*, 45(6):452-464.

Kritikos, T.M., DeVoe, E. (2018) Parenting on the homefront through military cycles of deployment. *International Journal of Birth and Parent Education*, 5(4):7-9.

Lake, A., Rosan, C. (2017) Being a military child: Guidance for engagement and early intervention with military families. *International Journal of Birth and Parent Education*, 4(3):26-28.

Lara-Cinisomo, S., Chandra, A., Burns, R.M., Jaycox, L.H., Tanielian, T. et al. (2012) A mixed-method approach to understanding the experiences of non-deployed military caregivers. *Maternal and Child Health Journal*, 16:374-384.

Lieberman, A.F., Van Horn, P. (2013) Infants and young children in military families: A conceptual model for intervention. *Clinical Child and Family Psychological Review*, 16:282-293.

Lincoln, A.J., Sweeten, K. (2011) Considerations for the effects of military deployment on children and families. *Social Work in Health Care*, 50(1):73-84.

MacDonell, G.V., Bhullar, N., Thorsteinsson, E.B. (2016) Depression, anxiety, and stress in partners of Australian combat veterans and military personnel: A comparison with Australian population norms. *PeerJ - Life and Environment*, 4:e2373.

Mansfield, A.J., Kaufman, J.S., Marshall, S.W., Gaynes, B.N., Morrissey, J.P. et al. (2010) Deployment and the use of mental health services among U.S. Army wives. *New England Journal of Medicine*, 362(2):101-109.

Mindell, J.A., Li, A.M., Sadeh, H., Kwon, R., Goh, D.Y.T. (2015) Bedtime routines for young children: A dose-dependent association with sleep outcomes. *Sleep*, 38(5):717-722.

Nolan, M., Misca, G. (2018) A review of coping strategies, parenting programmes and psychological therapies available to military parents with children under 5. *International Journal of Birth and Parent Education*, 5(4):10-14.

Office for Standards in Education (Ofsted) (2011) *Children in Service Families: The Quality and Impact of Partnership Provision for Children in Service Families*. Ref: 100227. London: Ofsted.

Osofsky, J.D., Chartrand, M.M. (2013) Military children from birth to five years. *The Future of Children*, 23(2):61-77.

Palmer, C. (2008) A theory of risk and resilience factors in military families. *Military Psychology*, 20:205-217.

Schaetti, B.F. (2002) Attachment theory: A view into the global nomad experience. In Ender, M.G. (Ed.) *Military Brats and Other Global Nomads: Growing up in Organisation Families*. Santa Barbara, CA: Praeger Publishers: 103-119.

Waliski, A., Bokony, P., Kircchner, J.E. (2012) Combat-related parental deployment: Identifying the impact on families with preschool-age children. *Journal of Human Behavior in the Social Environment*, 22(6):653-670.

18 A note on education and support for parents of twins

A mother who had given birth to twins commented that being part of the group of women who had met at antenatal classes had 'made this year bearable'. She explained this in terms that specifically referred to her mental health: 'I think if I hadn't had them, I would have needed something else to keep me sane'.
(Personal communication to the author in the course of her research)

Educators may prefer to include mothers and fathers expecting two babies in their regular groups to avoid their feeling that having twins lies outside the normal experience of the transition to parenthood. However, educators may also feel that the challenges these parents face require more time for reflection than is available in a standard group and therefore, that dedicated early parenting education is preferable. If twins' parents attend regular groups, there is, in fact, little that they need to know that isn't relevant to, or different from, what the other parents in the group need. Twin babies are more likely to be premature than singletons but it is helpful if *all* parents have given some thought to how their plans would be affected if their baby came early. In relation to infant feeding, the educator can acknowledge the challenges that parents may face if a baby is born prematurely or is of low birthweight and therefore not able to breastfeed straight away, but suggest that more information can come later if and when required.

Twin babies may also need to be born by caesarean section, although this is less common following the findings of the Twin Birth Study (Asztalos et al., 2016:abstract) which demonstrated that 'planned cesarean delivery provides no benefit to children at 2 years of age compared with a policy of planned vaginal delivery in uncomplicated twin pregnancies between 32–38 weeks' gestation where the first twin is in cephalic presentation'. While it remains more likely that twins will be born surgically and will need extra care in hospital, these eventualities could arise for any parents and discussion of the importance of building a relationship with babies who are in the Special Care or Neonatal Intensive Care Unit are relevant to everyone.

> If twins' parents attend standard early parenting groups, there is, in fact, little that they need to know that isn't relevant to, or different from, what the other parents in the group need.

Couple relationship

Even more than couples expecting one baby, couples expecting two need to spend time discussing how they will prioritise and divide the care of the babies and the household chores between them. The same discussions and activities as described in Chapter 11 will be highly relevant. So will an emphasis on maintaining positive mental health. Mothers and fathers expecting twins need time to identify for themselves and each other the activities in their lives which are a key component of their positive mental health and discuss how these can be continued, at least occasionally, after the twins are born. It is extremely important that early parenting education should enable fathers/partners to practise babycare skills as their help will be vital from the moment the babies are born, and the degree to which the couple pull together and are both involved in caring for their twins is likely to be highly influential in terms of their satisfaction with their relationship.

Breastfeeding twins

Bennington (2011:194) notes that, 'virtually all mothers can breastfeed one or more infants, provided that they have correct information and the support of their family, the health care system, and society at large'. As with other parents, there is only so much information that parents expecting twins can take in during pregnancy, and this is particularly so with regard to breastfeeding. The aim of early parenting sessions is to provide enough information about infant feeding to enable parents to make a choice about how they will feed their babies, to introduce key skills and, most importantly, to signpost them clearly to resources available to support them as soon as the babies are born and in the first weeks.

Practising different ways of holding a baby for breastfeeding is helpful for couples expecting twins as it is for other parents in the group. Many twins' mothers find that, until they become confident in breastfeeding, it is easier and quicker to feed the babies separately. This enables them to concentrate on each baby's attachment at the breast and also to give each baby individual time. Twins' mothers can therefore try out positions for holding one baby at the breast, and then for positioning two babies using the 'double football' hold, the 'double cradle' hold or combining the two with one baby being tucked under the mother's arm and the other cradled at the breast (Flidel-Ramon & Shinwell, 2002).

Other members of the family who will be involved in supporting the twins' parents after their babies are born should be invited to attend the breastfeeding/infant feeding session (or every session). Grandparents are probably the people most likely to be called upon to help the new family. They may be doubtful as to whether it is possible or desirable to breastfeed two babies, and enjoy learning about how successful breastfeeding can be achieved and what support the parents will need.

Other members of the family who will be involved in supporting the twins' parents after their babies are born should be invited to attend the breastfeeding/infant feeding session.

Sleeping arrangements

Twins' parents will have some queries that are specific to them, such as how best to sleep their babies. Hayward et al. (2015:193) state that 'co-bedding [putting the twins in the same cot] promotes self-regulation and sleep and decreases crying without apparent increased risk'. There seem to be no dangers to twins sharing the same cot provided that appropriate bedding is used to eliminate the risk of suffocation, and the twins are placed on their backs. It may be that the babies sleep better when together, and are more likely to wake at the same time, making feeding them together easier and maximising the parents' time to rest. However, the decision whether to use one or two cots is, of course, entirely the parents'.

Sharing stories

Parents of twins will benefit from hearing about other couples' experiences in the early weeks and months with their twins, and the educator can invite a mother and/or father from the local Twins Group to visit. It may be important to choose a couple who can present a realistic, but balanced, view of parenting twins, and who enjoyed a positive experience of breastfeeding if that was their infant feeding choice. The educator can encourage the visitors to talk about topics that will be relevant to all the parents in the group, such as strategies for getting enough sleep, and topics particularly relevant to the twins' parents, such as whether to sleep the babies in the same cot or separately. The educator may also ask the visiting parents about their relationship with each baby, whether one baby has been 'easier' than the other, about the similarities and differences between the babies and each baby's preferences, and how they try to treat each child equally. The aim of these questions is to support the expectant parents to see each of their babies as an individual, rather than as 'one of the twins'. If twins' parents are not able to visit, the educator can find clips from YouTube of parents talking about their babies, or sections from books and magazines which tell stories that present a realistic, positive account of early parenthood with twin babies.

Support

An activity where parents brainstorm the different sources of support that they can access after the birth of their babies is especially relevant to twins' parents, and may elicit useful information from participants about venues particularly welcoming to twins that the educator her/himself may not have known about.

> More than anything else, it is vital for parents expecting twins to build a support network.

Perhaps more than anything else, it is vital for parents expecting twins to build a support network. The educator can signpost them to organisations especially for twins. However, it is also important if the parents are attending a standard early parenting programme, rather than one dedicated to twins' parents, that the educator encourages the group to arrange postnatal get-togethers in places accessible to the twins' parents, and to include them fully in any plans for meeting after the programme has finished. With encouragement, the singleton parents can think about how to ensure that the twins' mother and father do not become isolated from the rest of the group. Belonging to a group where the other parents have just one child helps 'normalise' the twins' family and the support it provides may be a lifeline in terms of the mother's and father's mental health, as illustrated by the quote at the head of this chapter.

Key points

- There is little that twins' parents need to know that isn't relevant to other parents in the group
- While twin babies are more likely to be premature than singletons, it is helpful for *all* parents to consider how they would manage if their baby came early and how they would build a relationship with him or her in the Special Care Unit
- It is even more important for twins' parents than singleton parents to reflect on how they will nurture their own relationship across the transition to parenthood and maintain positive mental health

- Parents of twins should be invited to attend the breastfeeding session (or, indeed, all sessions) with other members of their family who will be involved in supporting them after their babies are born
- Hearing other couples' experiences in the early weeks with their twins is important for ensuring that parents expecting twins are realistically prepared
- Educators should strive to help parents expecting twins to build a support network

Note

In the Appendix are teaching activities, 'Exploring mental health', 'Myths and realities about babies', 'Feeding stars', 'Finding time for each other' and 'What do you want for your baby? What does your baby need?', which may be useful in facilitating sessions for parents of twins.

References

Asztalos, E.V., Hannah, M.E., Hutton, E.K., Willan, A., Allen, A.C. (2016) Twin birth study: 2-year neurodevelopmental follow-up of the randomized trial of planned caesarean or planned vaginal delivery for twin pregnancy. *American Journal of Obstetrics and Gynecology*, 24(3):371.e1-371.e19.

Bennington, L.K. (2011) Breastfeeding multiples: It can be done. *Newborn and Infants Nursing Review*, 11(4):194-197.

Flidel-Ramon, O., Shinwell, E.S. (2002) Breast-feeding multiples. *Seminars in Neonatology*, 7:231-239.

Hayward, K.M., Johnston, C., Campbell-Yeo, M.L., Price, S.L., Houk, S.L. et al. (2015) Effect of cobedding twins on coregulation, infant state and twin safety. *Journal of Obstetric, Gynecologic and Neonatal Nursing*, 44(2):193-202.

19 A note on early parenting education for mothers and fathers from minority communities

It is hugely important to consider the underlying values of a community, along-side proven psychological parenting principles, when creating or adapting parent education programmes to ensure good outcomes and acceptability of group parenting programmes.

(Hussein et al. 2017:4)

In 2011, Dumas et al. claimed that early parenting education programmes were failing to meet the needs of mothers and fathers from minority communities owing to culturally and/or religiously incompatible content. It is to be feared that this situation has not greatly improved over the last decade and perhaps will only be effectively addressed when sufficient skilled birth and parenting educators have been trained from the communities themselves.

It is, of course, unintelligent and unhelpful to see all parents who come from, for example, a West Indian, African, Pakistani, Indian or other background, or who are Jewish or Polish, as being 'the same' and requiring something different from the majority population in terms of early parenting education. However, it is appropriate to ask whether some of these parents might shun a universal programme because certain aspects are uncomfortable for them, conflicting with their cultural or religious values. Some (but by no means all) parents who are Muslims will be unwilling to participate in groups that include both fathers and mothers; however, they might be happy to attend a programme for mothers only or fathers only. There are other issues which are fairly simple to resolve such as the day of the week on which sessions are held. Fridays, Saturdays and Sundays may not accommodate parents who are devout Muslims, Jews or Christians.

For educators who come from a secular background and whose lives are not shaped by religious beliefs and practices, it may be hard to understand the way in which religion permeates every aspect of the lives of those who are devout adherents of their faith. However, if universal early parenting education is to be truly 'universal', it needs to present its key messages in a variety of ways so that it can reach out to groups who feel that sessions which pay no attention to their culture or religious ideals are not what they want. Research by Davis et al. (2012) has noted that a programme may be evidence-based and robust in its theory of change, but if it is not culturally adapted, it will fail to attract and retain mothers and fathers from certain communities.

> When adapting a programme for a minority group, it is vital to identify and retain the core components or risk compromising the programme's effectiveness.

The work of Kumpfer and colleagues (2008) in reviewing the implementation of the Strengthening Families programme (https://strengtheningfamilies program.org/) across the world is useful in considering how best to adapt an early parenting programme for minority groups. Strengthening Families is a substance abuse prevention programme, originally designed for at-risk children aged six to twelve years, that offers fourteen family-centred skills training sessions. It has been successfully adapted for use in seventeen countries. Kumpfer and colleagues (2008:230) stress that it is vital 'to identify and retain the core components' of whatever programme is to be adapted or risk compromising its effectiveness. Cultural adaptations of the 'surface structure' of an existing programme will go some way to engaging and retaining parents. Surface adaptations include:

> *Adding culturally appropriate welcomes, blessings on the group, songs, stories, dances, exercises, examples, pictures, videos...*
>
> (Kumpfer et al. 2008:230)

However, Thomson et al. (2018) consider that surface adaptations are insufficient to meet the real needs of parents from minority communities. An alternative, therefore, to adapting an existing programme is to create a new one that is co-produced with the minority group in question. Hussein et al. (2017) argue that:

> *Involving the target population in the design of a new parenting programme gives ownership of the programme to the community and enhances its meaning, thereby yielding stronger results ... It may also be hypothesised that such programmes will draw on the deeper values described by Resnicow et al. (2000) forming a mechanism for change.*
>
> (p4)

Co-creation has been found to be a key element in reaching out to Indigenous people, such as the Māori of New Zealand. Keown and colleagues (2018) describe how a low-intensity, two-session group variant of the Triple P-Positive Parenting Program (www.triplep.net) was adapted for Māori parents of young children. This involved close collaboration with Māori tribal elders, practitioners as end-users of the adapted programme, and parents as consumers, in order to ensure that traditional Māori cultural values were incorporated. 'The culturally adapted program was associated with high levels of parental satisfaction' (Keown et al., 2018:954).

Co-creation of parent education programmes has been found to be a key element in reaching out to Indigenous people.

Early parenting education that is based on both the evidence from research into effective parent education programmes and on parents' cultural and religious values may encourage mothers and fathers to attend programmes which they would not attend without such a foundation. Scourfield and Nasiruddin (2014) have described religious adaptation of the Family Links Nurturing Programme (https://familylinks.org.uk/the-nurturing-programme) in order to target Muslim parents and have described how the programme was received by the fathers (and by their wives who attended a separate programme for women only). Adaptations included:

- Running the programme via single-sex sessions
- Using the community language
- Having facilitators from the same faith and culture as the fathers (and mothers)
- Using texts from *Qur'an* and *Hadith* to justify the content and 'messages' from each session of the programme
- Scheduling sessions at appropriate times and locations.

Religious teachings bolstered the core themes of the Nurturing Programme but nothing was removed. 'The intention [was] to preserve all the core elements of the original (secular) programme, but to package them for a Muslim audience with Islamic teachings that [were] compatible' (Scourfield & Nasiruddin, 2014:700). Participants were 'given examples from the life of the Prophet Muhammad to demonstrate that the proposed [parenting] strategies [did] not contradict Islamic principles' (Scourfield & Nasiruddin, 2014:701). If a female facilitator was co-facilitating a session for fathers, she left the room when sex was discussed, although, for all other topics, the fathers were quite happy to have a female facilitator from their own faith. The researchers felt that the adapted programme overcame the double alienation that Muslim fathers may feel if confronted with a secular programme centring on mothers.

Other programmes for Muslim families have adopted similar principles. The organisation Approachable Parenting, based in Birmingham, UK, is headed by a Muslim mother who is a midwife and counsellor. The organisation runs the 5 Pillars of Parenting programme to support mothers and fathers of children aged four to eleven and is described as drawing upon both psychological and Islamic principles in the same way that the Family Links Nurturing Programme does. It gives parents practical guidance and offers them tools that 'Muslim parents need to raise their children' and to enhance their skills to provide 'consistent value-based parenting in line with their own religious beliefs' (Islamic Relief, 2019). The 5 Pillars progamme employs interpreters, as do many health education programmes for minority communities. While invaluable in reaching out to parents, it is critical that interpreters are well briefed. Thomson et al. (2018) describe how trained interpreters should meet with facilitators prior to the programme to become familiar with its aims and content so that they are able to deliver alongside the facilitators at each session.

While not an early parenting programme, the approach used in the 5 Pillars of Parenting is clearly transferable to programmes that cover the transition to parenthood. The evaluation carried out by Thomson et al. (2018) concluded that its success lay in the balance of psychological theories with Islamic references and that the key attributes of the facilitators were, therefore:

- That they were Muslim (that is, self-identified with the Muslim faith)
- They were able to understand the key concepts of the programme
- They knew how to seek support when parents asked for clarification on Islamic concepts
- They had a recognised teaching qualification.

Continuous adaptation

There is little literature on the adaptation of early parenting education programmes based on Western culture and values for parents from other communities, be these faith-based communities or communities with different cultures, such as those of the Indigenous peoples of Australia and the First Nations peoples of Canada. Far more work needs to be done. The process of cultural adaptation is continuous (Kumpfer et al., 2008), and educators working with groups that have been poorly served by parenting education interventions need to seek regular feedback from those with whom they are co-creating programmes, the parents who attend the sessions, parents who don't attend and community leaders.

Key points

- Some parents may shun a universal early parenting programme because certain aspects conflict with their cultural or religious values
- It is vital to identify and retain the core components of any programme to be adapted or risk compromising its effectiveness
- 'Surface adaptations' to an existing programme may be insufficient to meet the real needs of parents from minority communities. An alternative, therefore, is to co-produce a new programme with members of the minority group
- Educators need to seek regular feedback from those with whom they are co-creating and leading programmes, including the parents who attend sessions, those who don't and community leaders

Note

In the Appendix are teaching activities, 'Exploring mental health', 'Myths and realities about babies', 'Feeding stars', 'Finding time for each other' and 'What do you want for your baby? What does your baby need?' which may be useful in facilitating sessions for parents from minority communities.

References

Davis, F.A., McDonald, L., Axford, N. (2012) *Technique is Not Enough: A Framework for Ensuring that Evidence-based Parenting Programmes are Socially Inclusive*. The British Psychological Society. Available at: www.researchgate.net/publication/268202768_Technique_Is_Not_Enough_-_A_Framework_for_ensuring_Evidence_Based_Parenting_Programmes_are_Socially_Inclusive (accessed 11 July 2019).

Dumas, J.E., Arriaga, X.B., Begle, A.M., Longoria, Z.M. (2011) Child and parental outcomes of a group parenting intervention for Latino families: A pilot study of the CANNE program. *Cultural Diversity and Ethnic Minority Psychology*, 17(1):107–115.

Hussein, H., Thomson, K., Roche-Nagi, K. (2017) Parenting programmes are not culturally relevant to many communities. *International Journal of Birth and Parent Education*, 5(1):3–4.

Islamic Relief (2019) *Approachable Parenting: Award-winning Parenting for British Muslim Families*. Available at: www.islamic-relief.org.uk/approachable-parenting-award-winning-parenting-for-british-muslim-families/ (accessed 11 July 2019).

Keown, L.J., Sanders, M.R., Franke, N., Shepherd, M. (2018) Te Whānau Pou Toru: A randomized controlled trial (RCT) of a culturally adapted low-intensity variant of the Triple P-Positive Parenting Program for Indigenous Māori families in New Zealand. *Prevention Science*, 19:954–965.

Kumpfer, K.L., Pinyuchon, M., Teixeira de Melo, A., Whiteside, H.O. (2008) Cultural adaptation process for international dissemination of the Strengthening Families program. *Evaluation & the Health Professions*, 31(2):226–239.

Resnicow, K., Soler, R., Braithwaite, R.L. (2000) Cultural sensitivity in substance use prevention. *Journal of Community Psychology*, 28(3):271–290.

Scourfield, J., Nasiruddin, Q. (2014) Religious adaptation of a parenting programme: Process evaluation of the Family Links Islamic Values course for Muslim fathers. *Child: Care, Health and Development*, 41(5):697–703.

Thomson, K., Hussein, H., Roche-Nagi, K., Butterworth, R. (2018) Evaluating the impact of the 5 Pillars of Parenting programme: A novel parenting intervention for Muslim families. *Community Practitioner*, 13th March. Available at: www.communitypractitioner.co.uk/resources/2018/03/evaluating-impact-5-pillars-parenting-programme-novel-parenting-intervention (accessed 14 July 2019).

20 The way forward

Preconception education and support

Powerful 'teachable moments' for influencing parenting ... exist across the life course, not just during the antenatal or postnatal periods.

(Sher 2017)

Once a woman is pregnant and the decision to have a baby has been taken by herself alone, or with a partner, or she has become pregnant without any decision ever having been taken, the die has been cast for the baby she is carrying. While educators and clinicians can help her to achieve as positive a lifestyle as possible to support a healthy pregnancy, nine months may be too short a time to address deeply embedded problems around poor mental health, obesity, lack of exercise, lack of sleep, alcohol, tobacco and drug abuse. This isn't to say that education and support across the transition to parenthood are a waste of time; to say so would undermine the purpose and content of this book! However, if the aim of such education is, ultimately, to change children's life trajectory for the better, it should start long before pregnancy.

The future mother and father are, in fact, being prepared for parenting from their own birth onwards. The earliest relationships they have with their parents and principal carers create the template for how they will themselves parent when their time comes. If they have been the recipients of sensitive, responsive, nurturing early care, they will understand – at an instinctive level – how to provide the same kind of care for their own children. Education for parenting starts in the early childhood of each and every one of us.

Therefore, logic would demand that well before we start to replicate - consciously or unconsciously – our own experience of being parented, we should have the opportunity to learn about what babies need to thrive. There are three currently undervalued opportunities to shape the parenting of future mothers and fathers, and of their children on an inter-generational basis. These are at school, in adulthood prior to first conception and in between pregnancies.

Preconception education in school

As the school curriculum moves away from instilling facts into children and young people – obtaining facts is now so easy, there's no need to memorise them – and towards helping students analyse information and acquire life skills to negotiate the complexities of the 21st century, there is a huge opportunity for parenting education to feature in every school. One such initiative is described here by Elizabeth Smith (2019), a midwife dedicated to improving breastfeeding rates in Scotland:

> *I wanted to start as early as possible, why wait until people are pregnant? … So we talked to young people in schools. Interactive sessions with all age groups led to a relaxed atmosphere for open and honest conversations. We did a whole school approach, speaking to every year group, along with their teachers. We'd told the teachers that they were welcome to leave us to it, but they all stayed. Many later said that they had learned enough that they could be involved in helping to deliver future sessions.*
>
> *The project allowed us to test and develop sessions for nursery, primary and secondary schools. And the work is now being taken forward as part of a national programme to introduce children and young people to breastfeeding and discuss early nutrition.*

Parenting education in schools enables young people to think about some of the most important decisions they will ever have to make: Do I want to become a mother/father? How do I avoid becoming a parent before I want to, or at all? What can I do now and in the future to help me be the best possible mother or father and give my babies the best possible start in life? Who can help me have a healthy pregnancy and be a good parent?

Preconception education prior to the first pregnancy

A second opportunity to provide meaningful education and support for early parenting comes in adulthood, prior to the first baby being conceived. Stranger Hunter (2017) argues that preconception education should be the responsibility of primary care. Her One Key Question (OKQ) initiative in the USA attempts to ensure that every woman of childbearing age attending her GP surgery for what-ever reason is asked whether she would like to become pregnant in the next year. According to whether her answer is 'yes', 'no', 'unsure' or 'OK either way', she can be directed to appropriate contraceptive services or to counselling, education and support to help her achieve a healthy pregnancy.

> *OKQ is therefore an entry point to offer patient-centered, evidence-based contraception care for women who do not want to become pregnant, and*

comprehensive preconception/interconception care for women who desire pregnancy.

(Stranger-Hunter 2017:21)

OKQ is particularly relevant to women facing profound challenges in their lives, such as drug dependency and alcohol abuse. Services not only need to support them in tackling their addiction, but also help them make choices about avoiding pregnancy, or about treatment options if they intend to embark on a pregnancy.

Preconception education in between pregnancies

Interconception education is another precious opportunity for education for birth and early parenting. The woman and her partner now have lived experience to draw upon when reflecting on how they would like their next baby to be born and how they would like to parent him or her. The opportunity to make changes to ensure a healthy future pregnancy starts immediately after the birth of the previous baby. Therefore, providing education for couples who are *considering* having another baby helps them embark on the next pregnancy in the context of a healthy lifestyle, a healthy relationship and having learned more about the nurture of very young children.

Political will

While initiatives to secure better pregnancies and parenting for the next generation of babies are laudable, their impact will be limited if they remain local and dependent on the drive and commitment of individual practitioners. All practitioners who understand the importance of education and support for early parenting must accept the responsibility of communicating with politicians and policy makers in order to increase their understanding of the need to ensure that all future parents – young children, adolescents, parents expecting their first baby and parents planning on having another baby – appreciate the importance of the 'critical 1000 days'. With political will and motivated, educated practitioners, preconception education for early parenting should become universally available.

References

Sher, J. (2017) Making preconception health, education and care real. *International Journal of Birth and Parent Education*, 4(4):4–8.

Smith, E. (2019) Being a catalyst for change. Available at: www.qnis.org.uk/blog/being-a-catalyst-for-change/ (accessed 27 August 2019).

Stranger Hunter, M. (2017) 'Would you like to become pregnant in the next year?' The One Key Question© initiative in the United States. *International Journal of Birth and Parent Education*, 4(4):19–22.

APPENDIX

Teaching and learning activities
(These activities originally appeared in the *International Journal of Birth and Parent Education*. Reprinted here with permission.)

Perceptions of labour and birth

Mothers and fathers often come to antenatal programmes with preconceived ideas about labour and birth based on what they have heard from friends and family members, seen in the media – films, television, newspapers and magazines – and, of course, learnt from the internet. These ideas may be inaccurate and can be frightening. Voicing their fears and discovering that they are not the only ones to feel anxious can be a relief, and finding out that there are things they can learn and do to enhance the birth and make the experience their own are empowering and reassuring. How can educators debunk some of the 'hype' around birth and help mothers and fathers start to understand the physical and emotional process and what they can do to help themselves?

Labour and birth – dream versus media portrayal

This activity can be introduced early in an antenatal programme in preparation for an agenda-setting exercise, or later in the programme, as a means of exploring perceptions of pain in labour and of birth.

Aims

- To support self-efficacy by helping mothers and fathers analyse the representations that surround them of labour and birth
- To support parents in exploring their options for their own labour and birth.

Learning outcomes

As a result of engaging with this activity, mothers and fathers should be better able to:

- Identify some of the prevailing 'myths' around labour and how the media's presentation of birth is often unhelpfully negative or unrealistically 'glossy'
- Develop realistic ideas about the range of experiences that they may have or wish to have
- Identify tools and strategies to help them approach labour and birth with confidence and empower them to shape their own birth
- Demonstrate self-efficacy.

Method

At the top of a piece of flipchart, draw or attach a picture of a heavily pregnant woman or woman in labour (with her partner or other support person).

To one side of the image, write 'Dream Birth' and on the other side, 'Media Birth' (Figure App.1).

On sticky notes, ask group members to write one or two words to summarise their 'dream' or imagined labour and birth, and on sticky notes of a different colour, ask them to write a word or two about how they have seen labour and birth portrayed in the media. Ask each person to place her or his sticky notes on the appropriate side of the flipchart.

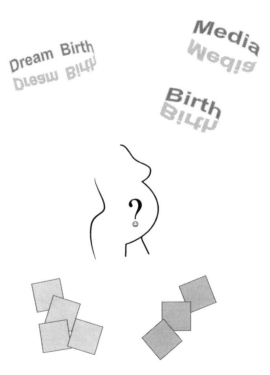

Figure App.1

Ask for a volunteer to read out the sticky notes and highlight the fears and hopes that group members share in common.

Facilitate a discussion to explore the 'myths' and start to develop more realistic expectations of labour and birth.

Questions to support discussion

- Do you have any family stories about labour and birth?
- Do you think 'difficult births' portrayed in the media are part of the reason for some women choosing not to have a baby at all, or becoming overly fearful of giving birth?
- What do you think directors of programmes such as *One Born Every Minute* are trying to 'say' or achieve?
- Why do we give such weight to scare stories?
- How do you find high-quality, evidence- based information on the internet?

Final activity

Draw a 'bridge' from the media birth to the dream birth and ask group members what they feel they might be able to do to achieve a fulfilling and empowering birth experience. Ask what topics and skills they might like to cover in the antenatal programme that would help them feel more confident and prepared. Explain how the programme will develop their understanding of the process of labour and birth and equip them with strategies for coping.

Note

This activity could introduce an agenda-setting activity, and lead on to exploration of other topics such as:

- How fear and anxiety influence the perception of pain
- The fear-tension-pain cycle (Figure App.2) and how understanding the process of labour and birth and practising skills for coping with the intensity of contractions can break into the cycle
- Importance of relaxation
- Practising relaxation activities
- Positive birth stories.

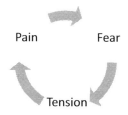

Figure App.2

As with many teaching and learning activities found in antenatal programmes, this one is a synthesis of ideas used by many practitioners. By adapting it to the needs of your own groups of mothers and fathers, and your own facilitation style, you can develop it further and make the activity your own.

(Prepared by Shona Gore, Consultant Perinatal Educator and Executive Editor of the *International Journal of Birth and Parent Education* and Kay Cram, Birth and Parent Educator, UK)

Breathing/practice contraction

Women gain confidence and a sense of control from having a 'toolkit' of strategies to help them manage the sensations of labour. This activity can demonstrate the benefits of using breathing awareness, movement and massage. Childbirth educators can help women and their partners to make sense of labour by acknowledging pain and enabling women to work with it as part of a normal birth experience. Practising increases the likelihood that parents will use the skills they have learned in the antenatal sessions.

Aim

- To increase parents' ability and confidence to manage labour.

Learning outcomes

As a result of participating in this activity, parents will be able to:

- Demonstrate a pain-coping technique which combines breathing, movement and partner support
- Choose an upright position which feels comfortable
- Compare different methods for managing the sensation of contractions.

Description

1. Ask the group to sit doing absolutely nothing while you time a minute.
   - Ask the group how that felt.
2. Time another minute and ask the group to count their breaths – breathing in and out counts as one breath.
   - Ask the group how that compared. (The majority of the group will usually say it felt a shorter length of time.)
3. Invite the pregnant women to choose a position which might be comfortable for labour or birth. Birth partners can offer massage or be a physical support to lean against. Ask all group members to count their breaths again while you time another minute, and invite the pregnant women to sway/move if they feel comfortable to do so.
   - Again, ask the group how that compared. (At this point, the parents usually say they took fewer breaths during the third minute than they did in the previous timed minute.)

Group discussion

Ask the parents why the third activity felt different and how this relates to labour. They will often say that, because they had breathing, positions and movement to focus on, the time went more quickly – they weren't just sitting there waiting for the 'contraction' to end. They might also say that the movement and massage enabled them to focus more easily on their breathing pattern, resulting in longer, slower and fewer breaths.

At the end of this activity, remind parents that they are more likely to use and benefit from the coping skills they learn if they practise them at home. Practising breathing techniques and labour positions for even a minute every day can make them feel more familiar and therefore more accessible in labour.

Variation

Another option is, for the third minute, to ask parents to count down from the number of breaths they took in the second timed minute. For example, it they took nine breaths in the second minute, ask them to count down from nine in the third minute. They will usually find that they don't reach zero, making it clear that the tendency is to breathe more slowly in the third minute.

(Prepared by Virginia Campbell, Formerly Head of Education and Practice at NCT, UK and Charlotte Whitehead, Yoga for Pregnancy Tutor and Pathway Lead at NCT, UK)

Preparing for the realities of early postnatal life

Aim

- To prepare parents for the realities of the immediate postnatal period and the challenges those days and weeks might present.

Learning outcomes

As a result of this activity, parents will be able to:

- Make realistic plans for their first weeks as parents
- Draw on strategies for dealing with the challenges of early parenting
- Identify what support they might need during this time.

Activity

In a same-sex group (pregnant women or partners/non-pregnant women), participants are asked to look at pie charts which show a baby's feeding/sleeping patterns over the first two weeks of the baby's life.

Each pie chart shows a period of 24 hours and participants are presented with day 2 (Figure App.3), day 4, day 7 and day 14.

(The pie charts come from The Breastfeeding Network and are free to use if credited: www.breastfeedingnetwork.org.uk. They can illustrate the pattern of feeding of either a breastfed or bottle-fed newborn.)

The facilitator encourages a conversation about how every baby is different and how, in the early days, the baby will not be ready for a bedtime routine or feeding schedule.

S/he then invites the parents to imagine that the baby whose days are laid out in the pie charts is their baby, and to write an action plan for each day using a sheet of flipchart paper with a column for each day.

The flipchart sheet suggests various activities that they might need to include in their days (Table App.1):

When will you:

- *Sleep?*
- *Prepare food and eat?*
- *Have a shower/bath?*
- *Look after pets or take the dog for a walk?*
- *Do housework?*

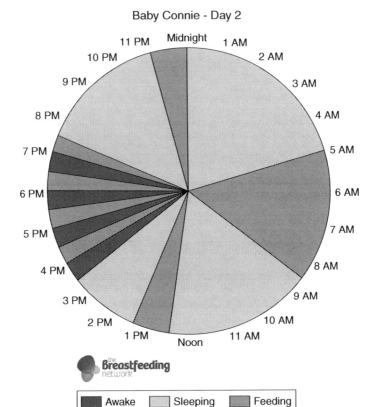

Figure App.3

- *Go shopping?*
- *Have visitors to the house?*
- *Go to visit people away from the house?*
- *Exercise?*
- *Work/return to work after paternity/maternity leave?*
- *Do hobbies/pastimes?*
- *Have social time?*

Discussion after the activity

Once the sheets have been filled, the facilitator invites a discussion. Some questions to help the discussion might be:

- How do these days differ from now, before the baby is born?
- Do you think you will have time to do everything?
- Are there things on the list that aren't important and could be dropped?

Table App.1

Day 2	Day 4	Day 7	Day 14	
				Using the pie charts to see when your baby will be awake / asleep / feeding, etc., work out what your days as a new parent might look like Think about when you might: Sleep Prepare food and eat Have a shower/bath Look after pets/take the dog for a walk Do housework Go shopping Have visitors to the house Go to visit people away from the house Exercise Work / return to work after paternity/maternity leave Do hobbies/pastimes Have social time

- What support networks do you have? Are there people who can help in a practical way by shopping, cooking, taking the dog for a walk, and so on?
- Every baby is different; this is just one example of how a baby might feed and sleep. Are there ways this baby could have fed/slept that would have made this task easier/harder?

Summary

This activity gives expectant parents the opportunity to think about the postnatal period in the context of their own lives and to start to make plans. It is also a means of starting an important conversation about support networks.

Further resources

- A list of the group's names, email addresses and mobile phone numbers (provided that everyone has consented to appear on the list). It is from other group members that parents are likely to find the best support.
- Contact details for infant feeding helplines and for local and national support organisations.

(Prepared by Vicki Sigston, NCT Antenatal Practitioner and Breastfeeding Counsellor)

Exploring mental health

Aim

- To promote wellbeing in mothers, fathers and significant family members during the first two years of a new baby's life.

Learning outcomes

By the end of this activity, participants will be able to:

- Identify activities that are important for their wellbeing and happiness
- Identify which activities are the most important in helping them feel positive about their lives
- Make some plans with their partner or significant family member(s) to be able to continue those activities in the first two years of the new baby's life
- Use breathing control and visualisation to achieve a relaxed state.

Activity

Ask your group what kind of things help them feel positive about their lives. Write everyone's responses around the circle (Figure App.4).

Split your group into smaller groups. You might choose to split them into single-sex groups to help both men and women to speak freely. Ask each group to discuss how they will continue to do some of the things they currently enjoy doing in the years before their babies go to pre-school.

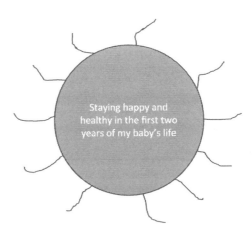

Staying happy and healthy in the first two years of my baby's life

Figure App.4

Then invite couples (the mother and the person accompanying her) to talk to each other about which activities in their current lives they would like to continue with while their baby is small, and how they could help each other to do this.

Conclude with a relaxation session, in which group participants are invited to use the out-breath to release tension from their muscles, followed by a script such as the story of the street sweeper which has a transferable message about taking labour one contraction at a time or life with a new baby one day at a time (www.goodreads.com/work/quotes/517524-momo).

Myths and realities about babies

Aim

- To enable mothers, fathers and co-parents attending an early parenting session to make decisions about their preferred parenting style based on accurate information about babies' needs.

Learning outcomes

This activity will enable group members to:

- Acquire up-to-date information about babies' need for nurture
- Identify commonly held misconceptions about babies' development
- Decide what toys they want for their baby and toddler
- Make decisions about when and how to develop a sleep routine with their babies and toddlers
- Understand how they can stimulate their babies' development by interacting with them.

Resources needed

Nine pieces of card, with one of the following statements printed on each:

1. Babies become spoilt and demanding if they are given too much attention.
2. When babies' needs for love and comfort are met, they will be calmer and grow up to be more confident.
3. It's important to get babies into a routine as this makes your life easier.
4. Young babies are not capable of learning a routine. Responding to their cues for feeding and comfort makes babies feel secure, so they cry less, which makes your life easier too.
5. You should leave babies to settle alone so they learn to be independent.
6. When babies are left alone, they think they have been abandoned, and so become more clingy and insecure when their parents return.
7. Babies benefit from lots of toys to help them learn.
8. Looking at your face is the best way for babies to learn.
9. Talking, listening and smiling trigger oxytocin and help your baby's brain to grow.

(Reproduced from the Baby Friendly Initiative leaflet, *Building a Happy Baby*, available at: www.unicef.org.uk/Documents/Baby_Friendly/Leaflets/building_a_happy_baby.pdf)

Activity

Spread the statements on the floor or on a table and ask group members to decide which statements are myths and which realities (myths: 1, 3, 5, 7; realities: 2, 4, 6, 8, 9).

Prompt discussion with questions such as:

Do any of these realities surprise you?

Do you think any of these realities would surprise friends who have babies, or your own parents?

Do you think the realities make parenting easier or more challenging?

When and how do you think you could start to develop a sleep routine with your baby or toddler?

Key message

Emphasise that all parents are trying to build a loving relationship with their baby, and that responding to babies' distress, and meeting their need for comfort and nurture, will not make babies clingy and dependent, but, in fact, will help them to feel secure and therefore, keen to explore the world around them as they grow up.

Feeding stars

Helping parents-to-be understand, prepare for and even enjoy the unpredictability of life with a young baby is key to supporting them through the first months of motherhood and fatherhood.

The following activity is a very simple one that nonetheless opens up important areas for discussion.

Aims

- To enhance the resilience of mothers and fathers-to-be in their parenting role
- To create a strong link in parents' minds between feeding their baby and building a relationship with him/her
- To increase enjoyment of early parenting.

Learning outcomes

As a result of participating in this activity, it is intended that parents-to-be should:

- Understand the unpredictability of new babies' feeding patterns
- Use the opportunity that feeding their baby gives them to build a relationship with him/her
- Be able to suggest coping strategies relevant to their individual circumstances.

Materials needed

1. Seven strips of coloured card for each couple or each small group of group members (Figure App.5)

2. Lots of sticky-backed stars (Figure App.6).

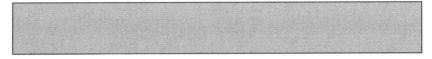

Figure App.5

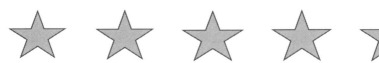

Figure App.6

Method

Give each couple, or each small group of parents, seven strips of card and a sheet of sticky stars. Ask them to place between six and twelve stars randomly on each strip of card.

After they have done this, explain that each strip of card represents a day of the week. On Monday, their baby may take six feeds with three clustered and the other three at longer intervals. On Tuesday, their baby may ask for twelve feeds so that the entire day is taken up with feeding. On Wednesday ... (and so on).

Ask

Do you feel that you understand why babies may have varied feeding patterns in the first months of life?

(Responses to this question reveal the level of knowledge of the group of the size of a baby's stomach, of the link between growth spurts and increased feeding and of their understanding that babies have no sense of 'routine' but only of 'need'.)

How does this make you feel about the first months of looking after your baby?

(Range of responses for discussion: worried; fearful; desperate; OK; we'll manage.)

What are the challenges?

(Range of responses: exhaustion; going mad; never getting anything done; frustration; being organised.)

What are the opportunities?

(Range of responses: time to get to know my baby; holding my baby close; talking to my baby; resting while my baby feeds; not feeling guilty about not doing housework!)

How are you going to cope?

(Range of responses: just accept that this is how it's going to be for a while; being organised with the household chores; feeding myself properly; trying to nap whenever I can; getting someone to help with everyday chores; getting out of the house.)

Conclusion

Summarise the challenges, opportunities and coping strategies that the group has thought of. Reassure them that the unpredictability of the first few months of their babies' lives will decrease as their babies grow, learn the difference between night and day and move towards a routine that suits them and their parents.

Acknowledgement

This activity is based on an idea of Judith Ockenden's from her chapter 'Antenatal education for parenting' (pp89-112) in: Nolan, M. (Ed.) (2002) *Education and Support for Parenting: A Guide for Health Professionals*. London: Baillière Tindall.

Finding time for each other

Aim

- To support the couple relationship in the early months of new parenting.

Learning outcomes

When they have completed this activity, couples will be able to:

- Anticipate and prepare for challenges to their relationship across the transition to parenthood
- Identify ways in which they currently support their relationship and some new ways of ensuring that they remain close once their baby is born.

Introduction

Explain that managing home, family and work commitments when there is a new baby often leaves partners struggling to find time for each other. It can be helpful to think in advance of ways of ensuring that your relationship remains strong.

Invite couples to work together for this activity. It is, of course, equally relevant to same-sex couples as to heterosexual couples. If a mother or father has come to the session unaccompanied, offer to work with him or her.

(If you are leading a session for women only, invite the women to work in small groups and then to continue the discussion with their partners at home.)

Give each couple (small group) a sheet of 'Relationship tips for new parents' (see below). Ask them to discuss:

- How many of these tips they currently use
- Which ones will be important for them after their baby is born.

Emphasise that this is a private discussion for each couple (group), and that they won't be asked to share what they've talked about. This may be a difficult activity for some couples, either because their relationship is struggling or because they're not used to having this kind of conversation. So set a manageable time limit – 'We'll take ten minutes for this'.

Relationship tips for new parents

Do you think the following tips will be useful to you after your baby is born? Can you put them into practice?

Commit to at least an hour of 'couple' time each week

That's time without children, friends or family members, when the focus is solely on each other. Put it in the diary and let it be a time you both look forward to. Couple time should be a high-priority event that doesn't get trumped for anything less than an emergency.

Celebrate anniversaries and significant dates

They're an opportunity to look at how you've grown both as individuals and as a couple, and remind you of the things that first brought you together. Try to do something special for your partner on these occasions; you don't need to spend money, just think of something that'll put a smile on his or her face.

Develop time management skills

If you want to spend time with your partner, but just can't find enough hours in the day, try to follow these four steps:

1. Plan ahead – ten minutes spent thinking about how to maximise your time over the day can save you hours.
2. Delegate – if someone can do something for you that will create time for your relationship, let them. It could be as simple as asking a friend to do some shopping for you on her way home from work.
3. Say no – simple, but effective.
4. Cut back on activities – you may enjoy them all but too many activities can put your relationship at risk; pick only the most important.

Don't bring up the negatives in your relationship on a date night

There's no quicker way to kill the mood and leave you feeling disconnected. If there are burning issues that need to be addressed, save them for a scheduled catch-up where the point is to focus on overcoming any obstacles in your relationship.

Do some homebuilding

While they might sound horribly like chores, decorating, gardening, cooking a meal or doing the food shopping together can actually build intimacy – and it gets things done in half the time!

Find a babysitter

Or if the budget won't stretch to one, put the baby to bed and schedule an 'at-home' date for later in the evening.

Signposting

At the end of the ten minutes, inform couples that if they want to do some more relationship work, they can visit meyouandbabytoo.co.uk where they can find an online relationship programme for new parents.

Acknowledgement

This activity is based on one devised by the charity, OnePlusOne: 'Finding time for each other'.

What do you want for your baby? What does your baby need?

Mothers and fathers who don't have much money (and those who do have) may enjoy an activity that helps them to distinguish between what a baby really needs and the things that new parents often buy, but aren't really needed!

Aim

- To support mothers and fathers to understand what a positive environment for their baby looks like
- To build understanding of the irreducible needs of babies.

Learning outcomes

By the end of this activity, participants will be able to:

- Identify items that are essential for a new baby
- Recognise that some items appeal to mothers and fathers but aren't necessary for babies
- Draw on the friendship and knowledge of other parents who have limited financial resources.

Activity

This activity can be done either in the whole group provided it is not too large (say, six to ten people), or in small groups.

Place a 'naked' doll on the floor in the centre of the room. Ask group members to suggest all the things that this 'baby' needs. Acknowledge and affirm everyone's contribution.

Fill in Table App.2, displayed on a flipchart stand. Ask group members to choose in which column to place the things that they have agreed the baby needs.

Alternatively, if your group members are confident to fill in the sheet on their own, invite them to work in small groups (possibly single-sex), giving each group a piece of paper with the headings on.

Table App.2

What you want for your new baby	What your baby needs	Where you can get this

Notes

- The 'naked' doll may trigger strong protective emotions in group members and this needs acknowledging and affirming
- The list of items that mothers and fathers would like might include: rocking cradle, cot, top-and-tail bowl, activity gym, dresses, sailor suits, shoes, a range of 'educational' toys, baby bouncer, cuddly toys, sit-me-up baby nest
- The list of what the baby needs might include: babygros, vests, reusable nappies or packs of newborn disposable nappies, Moses basket (or some-where for the baby to sleep), bottles and sterilising equipment if the parents have decided to bottle feed their baby, a sling, buggy, sheets and blankets
- Group members will also identify that the baby needs: love, play, warmth, cuddles, talking to, safety and feeding
- The list of where items can be obtained enables group participants to share their local knowledge of where 'the bargains' are, and perhaps to exchange items with each other. They will also recognise that 'what the baby needs' either costs nothing or can be purchased for relatively little money.

Discussion

The facilitator can draw out the following points:

- Babies' needs are very simple – to be fed, kept warm, clean and safe, and loved
- The 'baby industry' is keen to sell all sorts of items to new mothers and fathers that babies don't need
- New babies, under three months old, don't need toys – they need to look at their mother's and father's faces and be held close, talked to, and responded to when they cry (signal that they have a need)
- Babies are very happy with second-hand items!

Managing angry feelings

Aim

- To support group members to explore and gain a deeper understanding of why they become angry, how anger affects their relationship with others and how they do or don't manage their angry feelings.

Learning outcomes

After participating in this activity, group members will be able to:

- Describe their personal triggers for getting angry
- Acknowledge how they react when angry and how other people react to them when they're angry
- Describe a couple of strategies for managing anger as a parent
- Describe coping strategies that they could teach their children for managing angry feelings.

Activity

This is a potentially 'charged' activity, so it's important to make people feel as safe as possible while undertaking it. It is an activity that would be appropriate after a group has been through the 'forming', 'storming' and 'norming' phases of development, and is now in the 'performing' phase.

Small-group work (in pairs)

Ask group members to work in pairs – with whoever they choose.

Explain that each person will have five minutes to talk, without being interrupted by the other person, about things that make her or him angry.

Time ten minutes, signposting when five minutes are up and the other person in the pair needs to have their turn to talk.

Group brainstorm

Place a flipchart sheet of paper on the floor and ask group members to describe how they or other people they know react when they are angry. Ask for both physical and emotional reactions.

Group discussion

Initiate a discussion on coping with angry feelings.
Use open-ended questions:

- Why do small children make parents feel angry sometimes?
- Can anger ever be positive in parenting?
- How do you know when it's not positive but has become destructive?
- Can you tell us any strategies you use for managing angry feelings?
- Do these strategies always work? Why don't they work sometimes?
- How do you think being angry with a small child affects the child?
- What would you like your child to learn about being angry and managing anger as he or she grows up?
- How do other parents help their children to manage angry feelings?

Small-group work (in pairs)

Invite each pair, in private, to share any insights about their own angry responses that they have gained from the discussion, and any coping strategies that they have identified for use in the future.

Summary

Acknowledge that this has been a difficult topic for discussion, but a very important one. Finding acceptable ways of dealing with anger and disappointment is important for children and is a skill that they will take with them into adulthood.

Resources

Have internet links and contact details to hand for organisations that can help parents when they're struggling, such as OnePlusOne, Cry-sis, NCT and local parent support groups.

General family budgeting

Aim

To enhance parents' competence and confidence to manage their financial affairs after the birth of a baby.

Learning outcomes

After participating in this activity, group members will be able to:

- Understand in detail what their income and expenditure are now and are likely to be following the birth of their baby
- Know ways to reduce their expenditure
- Seek advice if needed.

Activity

Invite group members to fill in the budget sheet (see below). Support each individual to complete it accurately. Discuss with each individual plans for reducing expenditure and managing finances following the birth of the baby.

Budget sheet

1. Choose whether to fill this in for a month, a week or a fortnight, depending on how you receive your main income/benefit payments.
2. Be honest.
3. No really – be very honest and include cigarettes/alcohol/pet food etc.
4. If you get a negative balance at the end, do not panic. There is help available, and the situation can be solved. It just means that you need to act now (and it's a really good job you did the exercise today rather than leaving it another month – so well done). Make an appointment at your local Citizens Advice. Take all of your paperwork with you. If there is post that you are scared to open, take that too and you can open it together. If you are feeling miserable and need to talk to someone right now about your feelings, call the Samaritans.
5. If you did this exercise and found a surplus, that's great, but you should still check your benefit entitlement now that there is a baby on the way/just arrived. Are you getting the correct maternity pay/paternity leave? When did you last check your energy tariffs?

Income	Weekly/ fortnightly/ monthly	Expenditure	Weekly/ fortnightly/ monthly
Salary		Mortgage	
(Salary - partner)		Rent	
Benefits		Service charges	
Child Maintenance Service (CMS) payments		Council tax	
Child benefit		Contents insurance	
		Buildings insurance	
		Water	
		Gas	
		Electricity	
		Oil/heating	
		Broadband	
		Home telephone	
		Mobile telephone	
		Public transport	
		Petrol	
		Car insurance	
		Car tax	
		Car maintenance/ repairs	
		AA/RAC	
		Food	
		TV licence	
		Toiletries	
		Nappies	
		Milk	
		Pet food	
		Vets' bills	
		Christmas and birthday gifts	
		Hobbies (including music downloads etc.)	
		Magistrates' court fines	

Income	Weekly/ fortnightly/ monthly	Expenditure	Weekly/ fortnightly/ monthly
		Maintenance payable to ex-partner	
		Cigarettes	
		Alcohol	
		Clothing	
		Shoes	
Total		Total	

Now make a list of your debts and current repayment agreements (if you have any). There is a big difference between priority and non-priority debts. Non-priority debt includes water, catalogue repayments, vets' bills, loans, bank overdrafts. Often, if things are very tight and you have sought help, these people will accept minimum payments and will sometimes even agree to write off the debt. You will need to get help to draw up a financial statement and it's really useful to have someone 'on your side' to negotiate. Speak to your local Citizens Advice who will do this for free.

Never pay for debt advice.

Quick fixes to save money fast

1. Plan your shopping using a menu planner; this reduces cost and waste.
2. Don't shop when you're hungry!
3. Find out when your local supermarkets mark down their items (this happens regularly, like clockwork, every night and every week).
4. Get your energy bills out. Go to www.energyhelpline.com and save a lot of money fast. As a rule of thumb, the best way to save money is to have both gas and electricity with the same provider, pay by monthly direct debit and go paperless with all your bill information online. Tariff deals change weekly!
5. Register for emails with www.money saving expert.com.
6. Have a clear-out. Now put aside an afternoon to sell your unwanted stuff on eBay.
7. Ring your satellite TV provider. Tell them you plan to cancel unless they can reduce your monthly bill. They usually will.
8. Make a note in your diary when your insurance is up for renewal – now put another note in your diary a couple of weeks before this date to remind you to ring around and check on deals.

9. If things are tough, ring the people you owe and tell them you need help. Get support for this (see above).

10. Check that you are claiming all you can. Unclaimed benefits are measured in the millions.

Finally, if you or your partner or a family member with whom you're living has mental health issues, ask your GP to complete a 'debt and mental health evidence form', available at http://malg.org.uk/resources/malg-mental-health-and-debt-guidelines/debt-and-mental-health-evidence-form-for-advisers-assisted-self-help/

This can be very persuasive in helping you get a debt management plan in place with suppliers of services.

(Prepared by Helen Knight, NCT Antenatal Practitioner and Citizens Advice Advisor.)

INDEX

Abriola, D. 27
adrenalin 61, 84
Akerman, R. 15
Albertson review (UK, 2012) 177
Alcorn, K.L. 97
anger 228-229
antenatal education 1-2, 3-4, 9, 11-12, 14, 28, 29, 37-39, 56
antenatal education programmes 28-29, 60, 150, 177, 207-212, 213-217, 218-222, 223-229, 230-233
An Unfair Sentence: All Babies Count: Spotlight on the Criminal Justice System (NSPCC & Barnardo's, 2014) 176-177
Approachable Parenting 200
Apurva, P. 177
Arriaga, X.B. 197
artwork 90-91
at-home parents, military families 184-185, **186**, 187-188; mental health 185, 189
attachment 12, 34, 35, 37, 140, 145-146
Axford, N. 198

babies 35; mental health 2, 13; prison 175, 176; stress 2, 44-45, 137-138, 139
baby brain 44, 135, 137-138, 139, 143
babycare 12-13, 120, 125, 213-215, 218-222, 226-227; fathers 12-13, 105, 109-113
baby development 2, 8, 26, 34, 42-44, 135-136, 143; communication 140; emotions 140-141; music 43, 142; reading 141-142

Ball, H.L. 148
Barlow, J. 37
Barnett-Walker, K.C. 123
Baston, H. 97
Begle, A.M. 197
Begley, A. 177
Belsky, J. 45, 121
Bennett, C.T. 9
Bennington, L.K. 193
Bergman, K. 44
Berry Brazelton, T. 26-27
Betrán, A.P. 55
Better Births (NHS England, 2016) 29
Better Evidence for a Better Start (UK Social Research Unit, 2016) 29, 63
Bhandari, N. 25
Bhutta, Z.A. 150
birth 3-4, 11, 55-59, 60-62, 72-74, 207-212; difficult 91-94, 102; environment 57-58, 59-60, 63, 76; interventions 11-12, 55, 56, 66-68, 73-74; normal 3, 12, 55, 56; tokophobia 84-87, 88-90, 94; *see also* birth stories
birth companions 62-63, 91
birth hormones 59; adrenalin 63, 84; oxytocin 57-58, 59, 91
Birthplace in England Collaborative Group 72, 75-76
birth stories 63-66, 79-81, 97-98
birth stories workshops 98-101
Blinn, M. 122-123, 125-126
Bokony, P. 189

Brady, S. 27, 28
BRAIN mnemonic 169
breastfeeding 25, 112-113, 147-154, 155-157; twins 193-194
Bringing up Children (The Scottish Government, 2012a) 27, 105, 110
Bronfenbrenner, U. 8, 14, 17-18, 23, 108; ecological model 16, *17*
Brown, A. 149, 150, 152, 156
Brown, J. 15
Buchan, J.L. 9
budgeting skills 169-170, 230-233
Burton-White, L. 8
Butterworth, R. 198, 200

caesarean section 3, 11, 55, 73-74; twins 192
calm breathing techniques 48
Camacho, L.A. 150
Campbell, V. 61
Campbell-Yeo, M.L. 194
Carr, G. 28
Changing Childbirth (Department of Health, 1993) 29
Chartrand, M.M. 187
child abuse 10, 15
childbirth *see* birth
childbirth educators 1-2, 4, 5, 11, 55
childbirth review 98-101
childcare 125, 203; military families 185, 186-188
child development 8, 26-27, 107, 112, 132, 140-141, 142-143
child welfare 10, 105
Clapton, G. 108
co-bedding, twins 194
COFACE Families Europe 3
Cogan Thacker, D. 142
Coleman, L. 122
communication 12, 37, 140
communities 15
contractions 11, 56, 57-58, 61, 68, 87, 89-90, 91, 179, 211-212
coping strategies 121-122
couple conflict 14, 120, 123-125, 130, 228-229

couple relationship 14, 119-123, 125-126, 193, 223-225
couvade syndrome 105
Cowan, C.P. 121
Cowan, P.A. 121
Cox, M.J. 123
Coysh, W.S. 121
creative work 90-91
Creedy, D. 97
crying 135-137, 139-140
cultural adaptations 198, 200
Curtis-Boles, H. 121

Dad Project, The 22, 110
dancing 38
Davies, L. 90
Davies, R. 152, 156
Davis, F.A. 198
Deave, T. 63
de Oliveira, M.I. 150
depression 44, 130, 168; postnatal depression 113-114, 120; same-sex couples 130; young mothers 161, 171
Devilly, G.J. 97
difficult birth 102; self-assessment of distress 91-94
Domoney, J. 13
Donkin, A. 15-16
dreams 39, 43
Drummonds, M. 15
Dumas, J.E. 197

early (part of) labour 60
ecological model 16, *17*
Edgecombe, G. 15, 27-28
emotional regulation 135, 137-139
emotions 140-141; baby development 140-141; military families 188
environment 2-3, 5, 8, 42, 43, 44-45; birth 57-58, 59-60, 63, 76
ex-prisoners 180

Fairbrother, N. 90
families 2-3, 4, 10-11, 15, 18, 23; military 184-189

Family Included 108
Family Links Nurturing Programme 199
family services 10, 11
Fancourt, D. 142
Fatherhood Institute, The 63, 107, 170
fathers 97, 104–112, 113–116; babycare
    12–13, 105, 109–113; birth companions
    62–63; birth environment 60, 63;
    breastfeeding 112–113, 151–152, 153–154,
    156, 157; home birth 79; labour 61, 63,
    111; mental health 3, 13, 113–114; partner
    support 107; pregnancy relationship 35,
    105–106; stress 63; twins 192; unborn
    babies 35, 37
Fathers Inside 177
fear of childbirth *see* tokophobia (fear of
    childbirth)
Feinstein, L. 16
female prisoners 175, 176, 180–181;
    ex-prisoners 180; mental health 175;
    parent education programmes 177,
    178–179, 180–181
first-time parents 13–14, 35, 75–76, 77,
    102, 120
Franke, N. 198–199

gay couples 129, 130
Gilmer, C. 9
Glover, V. 44
Glynn, P. 27, 28
Goh, D.Y.T. 187
Graham, N. 35
guided relaxation 46, 47, 48, 49–52
Gutman, L.M. 15, 16

Hajeebhoy, N. 25
Hanna, B.A. 15, 27–28
Hayward, K.M. 194
health inequalities 5, 6
Heazell, A.E.P. 35
Heming, G. 121
Henriksson-Macaulay, L. 143
Heyman, R.E. 120
Hogg, S. 136
Holzinger, D. 28

home birth 72, 74–79; birth stories 79–81
Horsfall, J. 97
Horton, S. 25
Houk, S.L. 194
Houlston, C. 122
Houts, R. 123
Hunt-Martorano, A.N. 120
Hussein, H. 198, 200

Iles, J. 13
Imdad, A. 150
Inglis, C. 98
insecure attachment 12, 37, 140
institutions 7, 25, 68, 165
interconception education 205
internet *see* online education
interventions 6, 11–12, 55, 56, 66–68, 73–74

Jackson, C.A. 15, 27–28
Janssen, P. 90
Johnson, D. 63
Johnston, C. 194
Jordan, B. 73

Karatzias, T. 177
Kelly, J. 121
Keown, L.J. 198–199
Kiernan, K.E. 16
Kingdon, C. 55
Kirchner, J.E. 189
Kotelchuck, M. 15
Kumpfer, K.L. 198
Kwon, R. 187

Labbok, M. 152
labour 1, 3–4, 11–12, 55–57, 60–61, 207–212;
    birth companions 62–63, 91; contractions
    11, 56, 57–58, 61, 68, 87, 89–90, 91, 179,
    211–212; early (part of) labour 60; fathers
    61, 63, 111; interventions 12, 55, 56,
    66–68, 73–74; partners 61, 63, 91;
    relaxation skills 46, 56–57, 60–61, 89
lesbian couples 129, 130–131
Letourneau, N. 9
Li, A.M. 187

Lincoln, A.J. 188
Lok, K.Y.W. 150
Longoria, Z.M. 197
loss, pregnancy-related 35
Lutter, C.K. 25

McDonald, L. 198
McKellar, L. 68
McVeigh, C.A. 15
Māori parents, New Zealand 198-199
male prisoners 175, 176; ex-prisoners 180;
    mental health 175; parent education
    programmes 177, 181
Malik, J. 120
Malin, C.K. 15
Marmot, M. 5, 15-16
maternal stress 2, 44-46
medical intervention *see* interventions
Mensah, F.K. 16, 198
mental health 132, 216-217; at-home
    parents 185, 189; babies 2, 13; fathers
    3, 13, 113-114; mothers 2, 13, 15; parents
    2-3, 13; pregnant women 44, 87;
    prison 175, 179-180; young mothers
    161, 167-168
Mental Health Foundation 179
midwives 23, 68, 73, 74, 78
military families 184-189
Mindell, J.A. 187
minority communities 197-200
Mitcheson, J. 122
Mithen, S. 143
Moeller, M.P. 28
Mohiddin, A. 55
Molinuevo, D. 21-22
Mother and Baby Units (prison) 174, 176
mothers 14, 22; birth environment 59-60,
    63, 76; mental health 2, 13, 15; pregnancy
    relationship 36-37; social support 27;
    stress 2, 44-46; twins 192, 193; unborn
    babies 34-37
music 12, 37-38, 43, 142-143
Muslim parents 198, 199-200
mutual gaze 12, 140
Myles, M. 23, 104

Nasiruddin, Q. 199
National Parenting Strategy (The Scottish
    Government, 2012b) 15, 22
Nethery, E. 90
Newman, S. 15, 27-28
Newnham, E. 68
Nolan, M.L. 60, 61, 63
normal birth 3, 11-12, 55, 56

O'Connor, T.G 44
O'Donovan, A. 97
One Key Question (OKQ) initiative 204-205
online education 22, 51, 229
Opiyo, N. 55
Osofsky, J.D. 187
oxytocin 57-58, 59, 91

pain relief 56, 57-58, 67-68, 77, 78, 179;
    see also contractions; relaxation skills
Paley, B. 123
parental stress 2, 13, 44-46, 63
parent education 1, 3, 4-5, 7-8, 9-18, 21-22,
    34, 46, 58-59, 203
parent education programmes 7, 8, 10-11, 12,
    16, 17-18, 25-26, 29-31; breastfeeding 148,
    149, 150-151, 153, 155-157; couple conflict
    125; lesbian couples 130-131; military
    families 186-189; minority communities
    197-200; parenthood 120-122, 125; prison
    176-179, 180-181; relaxation skills 46-52,
    88-90; same-sex couples 130-132; twins
    192, 193, 195; young fathers 170-171;
    young mothers 162-170
parent educators 21, 22, 23-24, 26, 37
parenthood 7, 12, 13, 21, 120-122, 125
parenting education 6, 9, 21-23, 24, 25-26,
    204-205
parenting educators 6, 29-31
parenting groups 22, 24, 28
parenting skills 9, 24, 25; babycare 12-13,
    120, 125, 213-215, 218-222, 226-227
parents 2, 7, 10, 12, 24, 203; mental health
    2-3, 13; stress 2, 13, 44-46, 63; twins 192,
    194-195
parent support 3, 119

partners 62-63, 98; breastfeeding 153, 154, 156, 157; home birth 79; labour 61, 63, 91; stress 2, 63; tokophobia 94; twins 192
partner support 105, 107
Patel, A.D. 143
Patrick, J.C. 97
Peel Report (UK, 1970) 73
Perkins, R. 142
picture books 142
Pincombe, J. 68
Pinquart, M. 22, 121
Pinyuchon, M. 198
poetry 51-52
positive birth stories 63-66
positive coping strategies 121-122
positive parenting 4, 9, 10, 12, 16, 18
postnatal depression 113-114, 120
postnatal education 149
postnatal support groups 101
posttraumatic stress disorder (PTSD) 98
poverty 13, 16, 17
Power, K. 177
preconception education 204-205
pregnancy 34-39, 42-43
pregnancy relationship 23, 34-37, 43, 44-45, 105-106; *see also* unborn babies
pregnant women 23, 42, 44-45, 203; mental health 44, 87; partner support 105, 107; pregnancy relationship 34-36; prison 174, 175, 177, 178-179; stress 44-46; unborn babies 36-37
prenatal education 34; breastfeeding 149, 156; fathers 112; interventions 66-68
Price, S.L. 194
Prins, M. 97
prison 174-176; mental health 175, 179-180; parent education programmes 176-179, 180-181
Prison Reform Trust 175
PTSD *see* posttraumatic stress disorder (PTSD)

Ramchandani, P. 13
reading 141-142
Reed, R. 98

relationship education 167
relationship learning 135-136, 140
relaxation skills 46-52, 88-90; guided 46, 47, 48, 49-52; labour 46, 56-57, 60-61, 89
Rijnders, M. 97
risks 75-76
Roberts, J. 15-16
Robinson-Smith, L. 148
Roche-Nagi, K. 198, 200
Rollins, N.C. 25
Rouhe, H. 87
routines 187
Rudzik, A.E.F. 148

Sadeh, H. 187
Saisto, T. 87
salutogenesis 25
same-sex couples 129-132
Sanders, M.R. 198-199
Sarkar, P. 44
Schlossman, S.L. 7
Schneider, D. 100
Schonbeck, Y. 97
schools parenting education 204
Scott, D. 27, 28
Scourfield, J. 199
Seaver, L. 28
secure attachment 12, 34, 37, 140
self-assessment of distress 91-94
self-help skills 57, 60-61, 89-90, 101; *see also* relaxation skills
Shanker, S.G. 9
Sharman, R. 98
Shepherd, M. 198-199
Sher, J. 22, 25, 143
Shochet, I.M. 97
Simkin, P. 97
singing 12, 37-38, 43, 142
Slep, A.M.S. 120
Smith, A. 22, 37, 46, 47, 49
Smith, D. 7-8
Smith, E. 204
Smith, H.L. 7-8
social inequalities 15-16

social support 14-15, 28-29, 132; ex-
  prisoners 180; twins' parents 195; young
  mothers 170
Stephens, L. 35
Stoll, K. 90
story telling 63-66, 79-81, 97-101,
  194-195
straightforward vaginal birth 3, 12, 55, 56
Stranger-Hunter, M. 204-205
Stredler-Brown, A. 28
Strengthening Families programme 198
stress 13, 15; baby 2, 44-45, 137-138, 139;
  fathers 63; mothers 2, 44-46; partners
  2, 63; pregnant women 44-46; unborn
  babies 44-45
stroking 12, 38
surface adaptations 198, 200
Sweeten, K. 188
Swift, E.M. 90

Tarrant, M. 150
Tedstone, A.E. 15-16, 150
teenage mothers 160-161, 162-171
Teixeira de Melo, A. 198
Temmerman, M. 55
Teubert, D. 22, 121
Tew, M. 73
Thomson, K. 198, 200
Toivanen, R. 87
tokophobia (fear of childbirth) 84-87,
  88-90, 94
touch 38
traumatic labour 91-94; birth stories 97

Triple P-Positive Parenting Program 199
Tully, K.P. 152
Twin Birth Study 192
twins 192-195

UK Social Research Unit 29, 63
unborn babies 9, 23, 34-39, 42, 43-44;
  communication 37; dancing 38; dreams
  39; music 142; singing 37-38, 142; stress
  44-45; stroking 38; touch 38; *see also*
  pregnancy relationship
upright positions 61

vaginal birth 3, 11, 55, 56
Van Der Pal, K. 97
Verbiest, S. 15
very young children 9, 10, 137
visualisation 50

Waliski, A. 189
Welch, G.F. 143
Whiteside, H.O. 198
Wojcieszek, A. 35
Wong, K.L. 150
Woolston, C. 177
Wouk, K. 152

Yakoob, M.Y. 150
young fathers 170-171
young mothers 160-161, 162-171; depression
  161, 171; mental health 161, 167-168
YoungMumsAid 162
Young Mums Together 167

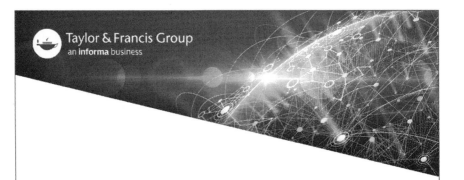